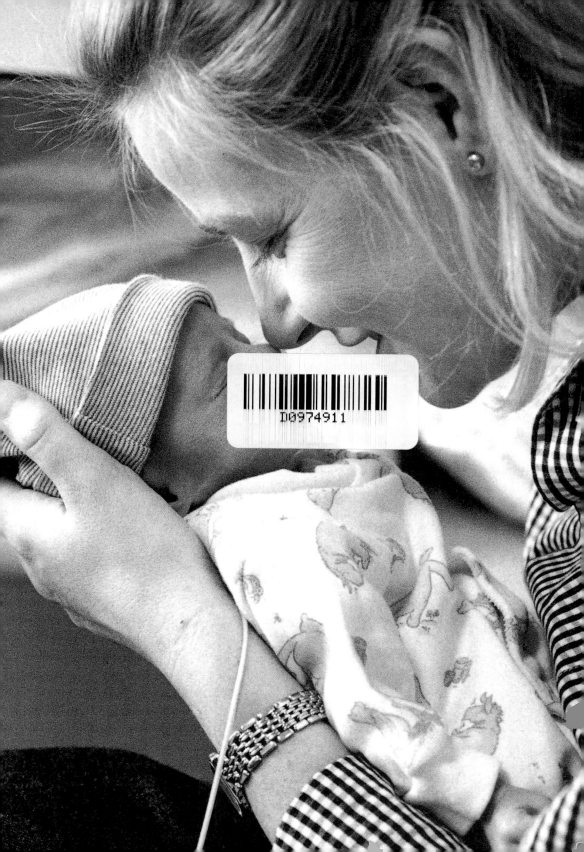

D0974911

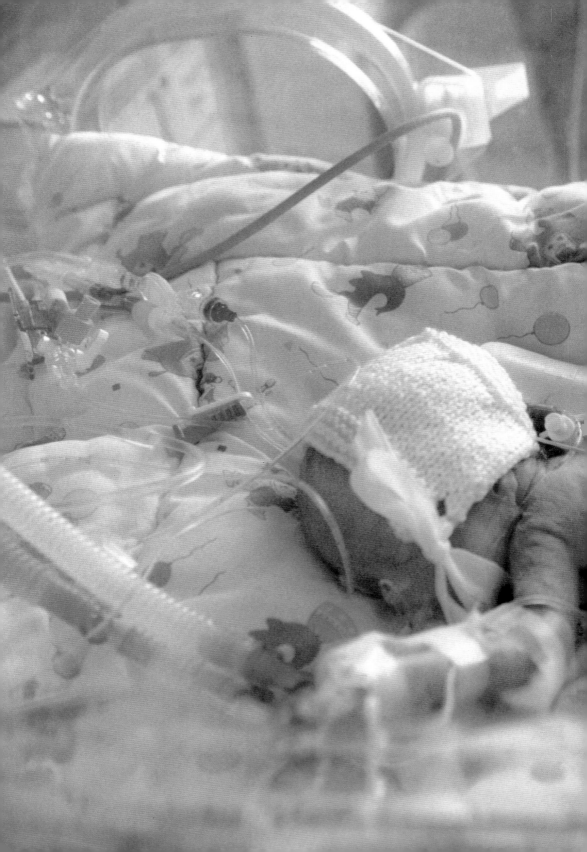

Your premature baby

the first five years

Nikki Bradford

*photographs by
Sandra Lousada*

FIREFLY BOOKS

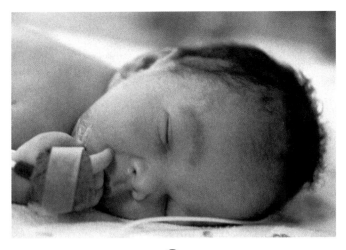

A Firefly Book

Published by Firefly Books Ltd., 2003
Copyright © Frances Lincoln Limited 2003
Text copyright © Nikki Bradford 2003
Photographs copyright © Sandra Lousada 2003
except for those otherwise indicated
Foreword copyright © Jonathan Hellmann 2003

First Printing

National Library of Canada
Cataloguing in Publication Data

Bradford, Nikki
Your premature baby: the first five years / Nikki Bradford;
photographs by Sandra Lousada.
Includes bibliographical references and index.
ISBN 1-55297-655-6 (pbk.)
1. Infants (Premature) 2. Infants (Premature)—Care.
3. Infants (Premature)—Development. I. Title.
RJ250.3.B73 2002   618.92'011   C2002-903166-4

Publisher Cataloguing-in-Publication Data
(Library of Congress Standards)

Bradford, Nikki.
Your premature baby: the first five years / Nikki Bradford;
Sandra Lousada. –1st ed.
[280] p. : ill. , col. photos ;   cm.
Includes bibliographical references and index.
ISBN 1-55297-655-6 (pbk.)
1. Infants (Premature). 2. Infants (Premature)—Care.
3. Infants (Premature)—Development. 4. Child rearing.
I. Lousada, Sandra. II. Title.
618.92/011   21   RJ250.B73   2003

Published in Canada in 2003 by
Firefly Books Ltd.
3680 Victoria Park Avenue
Toronto, Ontario
M2H 3K1

Published in the United States in 2003 by
Firefly Books (U.S.) Inc.
P.O. Box 1338, Ellicott Station
Buffalo, New York
14205

Printed in Singapore

DISCLAIMER
This book is intended to be a guide for parents who wish to understand more about their
baby's condition and is not intended to replace the advice of a medical practitioner.
Medical advice should always be sought before undertaking any form of treatment and it is noted that
advances in medical science or changes in medical practice may result in information contained in
this book becoming out of date. The publishers and author assume no liability or responsibility
for any damages resulting from the use of or reliance upon the information contained herein.

contents

Editor's Note: We have adopted the convention of calling the baby "he" in one chapter, "she" in the next.

foreword

The days of neonatal medicine, in which the parents of sick infants were passive bystanders and tacitly accepted physicians' decisions regarding medical interventions for their newborn infants are hopefully over. Today, physicians are expected to provide as much information as possible to parents, explaining it clearly and putting it into context so that parents can work together with the doctor to make decisions about their baby.

But communication, by its very definition, is the act of *exchanging* information, and so this means that parents too have a responsibility—to inform themselves as best they can about their baby's condition. The more information parents have, the better they will be able to deal with the concerns inherent in having a premature baby. Parents are important partners in the care of their baby: this is not just a cliché but an essential component to starting out the right way on the journey their premature baby is taking them on.

This book is a good guide to the journey. It is written to offer comfort and common sense, but more than that, its goal is to inform parents, to show them how they can participate in their baby's care as part of a team of physicians, residents, nurses and technicians. There is so much "information" available today that it is important to find and use information that is reliable and considered. *Your Premature Baby* attempts to offer just that. It is meant to be used as a tool by parents as they work with their baby's medical team, with whom they share a singular goal: to give their baby the best possible start in life.

Dr. Jonathan Hellmann, MBBCh, FCP(SA), FRCP(C)
Associate Professor of Paediatrics
University of Toronto
Clinical Director
Neonatal Intensive Care Unit
The Hospital for Sick Children, Toronto

author's acknowledgments

This book would not have been possible without the following people, who gave so generously of their time, advice, experience and expertise.

Very special thanks to:

Dr. Anthony Michael Kaiser, Consultant Neonatologist at St. Thomas' Hospital, London, for his invaluable help, tireless encouragement and advice on the sections about premature babies' possible medical problems and what can be done about them. He read much of the manuscript standing up on the tube on his way home after long, hot, late days and nights at the hospital.

And to:

Andrew Whitelaw, Professor of Neonatal Medicine at the University of Bristol, Southmead Hospital, **Neil Marlow**, Professor of Neonatal Medicine at Nottingham University, and **Ros Jones**, Consultant Neonatologist, Wrexham Park Hospital, Slough, for their help and suggestions on the chapter on the outcome for premature babies as they grow up.

Professor Phillip Bennett, Imperial College School of Medicine, London, for his help with the section on possible causes of premature labor.

Professor Neil McIntosh, neonatologist and Professor of Child Life & Health at the University of Edinburgh, for his help in connection with his work on cerebral palsy and premature babies.

Dr. Jeanine Young, at the time of writing developmental care expert, author and Research Midwife at the Department of Child Health, Bristol, for her support and advice on all the developmental care issues, including positioning and premature babies' communication.

Geoffrey Chamberlain, Professor Emeritus at the Singleton Hospital, Swansea, and immediate past President of the Royal College of Obstetricians & Gynaecologists, for his suggestions for the section on possible causes of prematurity.

Susan Bewley, Consultant Obstetrician at St. Thomas's Hospital, London, for her invaluable suggestions and feedback for the section on possible causes of prematurity.

Tilly Padden, neonatal nursing sister, researcher, midwife and Senior Lecturer in Midwifery Studies at the University of Lancashire, for all her help with the chapter on *You and your family*.

Sandra Lang, Consultant in Infant Feeding to UNICEF and the WHO, specialist in breast-feeding/cup-feeding of premature babies, for her advice on feeding.

Lisa Hollis, Community Liaison Neonatal Sister at Kingston Hospital NHS Trust, for invaluable guidance on and contributions to the chapters on *How little you are* and *Time to go home*.

Bridgette Riley, Family Care Sister at Derby City General Hospital, and Head of the Neonatal Nurses Association's Special Interest Group of Community Neonatal Sisters for her help with *You and your family* and *Time to go home*.

Chrissie Israel, Research Sister, and Parent-Baby Interaction Advisor at Southmead Hospital, Bristol, for her help with *You and your family*.

Joan Ritchie, neonatal nursing sister at Southmead Hospital, Bristol, for her advice on feeding.

Alree Hunt, neonatal nursing sister at St. Thomas' Hospital, London, for all her input into the chapter on how being born early may affect your baby.

Kathy Sleath, neonatal nursing practitioner of the Hammersmith Hospital, London, for her pioneering work with kangaroo care in the UK, and her help with this section of the book.

Monica Yonge, neonatal sister at Kingston Hospital NHS Trust, for her help.

Anna Collett, neonatal senior staff nurse and co-ordinator of the breast-milk bank at Kingston Hospital NHS Trust, for her suggestions on feeding.

Angela Newton, neonatal sister at the Starlight Unit, Barnet Hospital, London, and **Julie Honeychurch**, senior neonatal nurse and former sister at Southmead Hospital, Bristol, for their invaluable advice on positioning premature babies.

Janet Venn, neonatal sister at Musgrave Park Hospital (at the Taunton and Somerset NHS Trust), for her advice on therapeutic touch, color therapy and massage for premature babies.

Jenni Thomas, Founder-Director of The Child Bereavement Trust, and Bereavement Counsellor at Wycombe General Hospital, for all her help with the chapter on grieving and the loss of a baby.

Clare Delpech, Founder-Director of the Association for Post-Natal Illness, for her help with the section on post-natal depression.

Pauline Woods, Co-ordinator of Kingston Hospital NHS Trust's charity Born Too Soon, for all her kindness, enthusiasm and invaluable help with many different aspects of this book.

Dr. Sarah Levine, Medical Officer at the Foundation for the Study of Infant Deaths.

BLISS, the premature baby parents' support charity, for their help with the chapter on *What happens now?* and for helpful suggestions as to which experts to approach for other chapters.

The Neonatal Nurses Association for kindly putting us in touch with some of their specialist members.

Mark Hollinsworth, Researcher at the Information and Statistics Division (Scotland) Common Services Agency for the National Health Service for freely donating his time to track down various hard-to-find statistics in several different chapters.

All the SCBU nursing staff at St. Thomas' Hospital, London; at **Kingston Hospital NHS Trust**, Surrey; and at **Southmead Hospital**, Bristol: for their invaluable suggestions on several chapters.

Ruth Hudson of The Health Visitors' Association, for her advice on normal developmental checks for babies, toddlers and children.

And in the United States:

Professor Peter Nathanielz, New York, for his encouragement and suggestions right at the beginning of this project.

Professor John McGregor, Head of Obstetrics & Gynecology at Colorado University, for his advice and vision regarding the chapter on possible causes of premature labor.

And, very importantly, to the many dozens of parents of premature babies, who helped with advice and suggestions based on their hard-won experience.

Special thanks to:

The **Born Too Soon Parents Support Group** in Kingston, based at Wellcare House, and **Pauline Woods**, who took such time and trouble to introduce us; **Caroline and Trefor Hughes-Jenkins**, whose triplets, Tom, Ben and Megan, were born at 29 weeks; **Ashleigh and Mike**, whose daughter, Scarlett, was born at 31 weeks; **Louise Fulgoni**, whose daughter, Gabrielle, was born at 24 weeks; **Meera**, whose son, Rohan, was born at 26 weeks; and **Catherine Gibson**, whose son, Mark, was born at 31 weeks. Grateful thanks and admiration also to **Jo and Robert Robinson** from Nottingham whose son, Gregor, was born at 29 weeks and to **Bettina and Clive Radford** from Liverpool whose twin girls, Susanna and Madeline, were born at 33 weeks.

Firefly Books extends particular appreciation to:

Dr. Jonathan Hellmann, MBBCh, FCP(SA), FRCP(C), for his expertise and considered opinion. Dr. Hellmann graduated from the University of Witwatersrand in Johannesburg, South Africa, in 1970, and took his fellowship training in Neonatology at Hershey Medical Center, Pennsylvania. In 1983 he was appointed to The Hospital for Sick Children, Toronto. From 1987 to 1994, he was Clinical Director of the hospital's Neonatal Intensive Care Unit, where he resumed the position in 2000. Dr. Hellmann is also Associate Professor of Pediatrics at the University of Toronto.

Sharyn Gibbins, RN, MSc,PhD, for her enthusiastic assistance. Ms. Gibbins is a Registered Nurse with 17 years' experience of caring for premature and sick infants, including extensive experience in pain management for high-risk infants. She is a Clinical Nurse Specialist/Neonatal Nurse Practitioner at Toronto's Hospital for Sick Children and Head of Interdisciplinary Research & Evidence-based Practice at Sunnybrook Women's College Health Sciences Centre, Toronto.

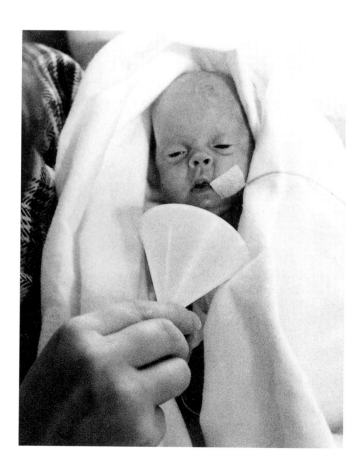

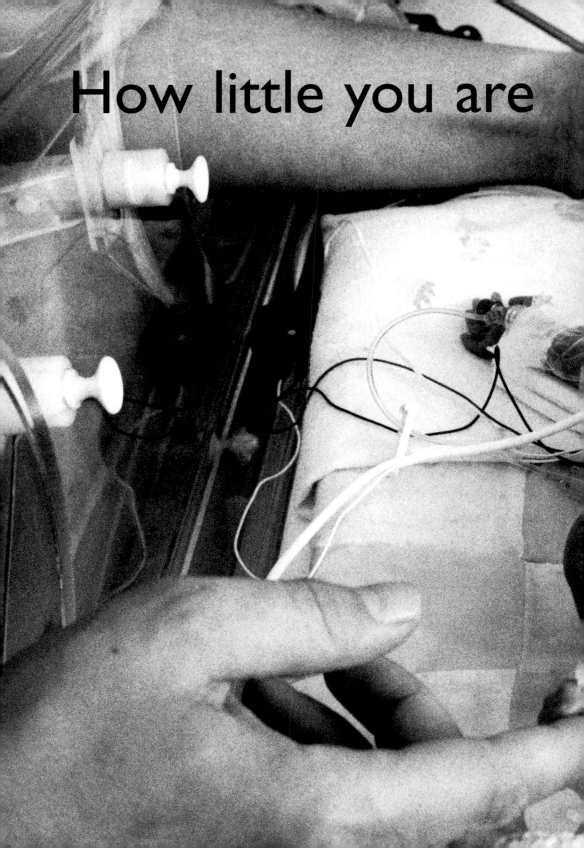

How little you are

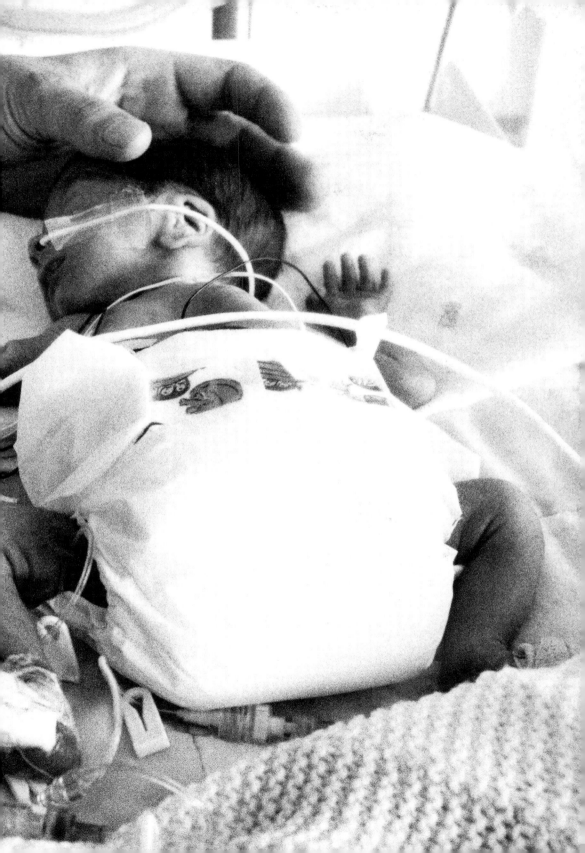

Your premature baby may not look like the one in the baby milk ads: in fact it's likely that he will temporarily look very different—sometimes disturbingly so, especially if he is very premature. He will also differ from a baby born at full term in what he can and cannot do for himself and how much help and medical support he may need for a while. These differences between the way your baby looks now and the mental image you had of the baby you'd hoped for may be upsetting, surprising or difficult to come to grips with, but it can help if you know roughly what to expect and the reasons for the differences. This chapter covers what babies of different degrees of prematurity may look like and what they may possibly be able to do or handle.

Born at 26 weeks: So small and skinny, and looking as if the lightest touch will bruise her.

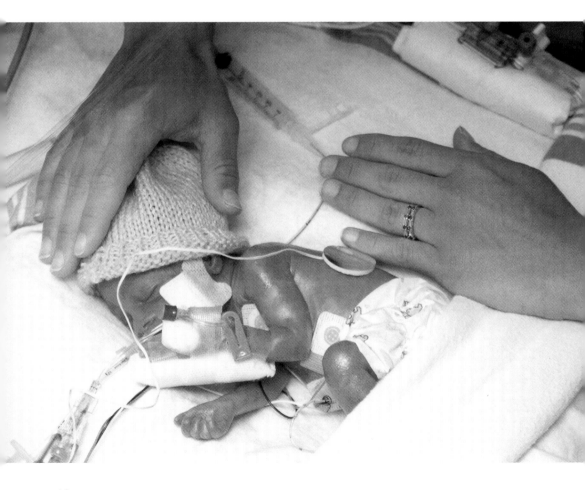

What does that word mean?

Medical staff may use terms that you have not heard before or whose technical meanings are unfamiliar:

Premature/preterm/prem baby:
a baby born before spending 37 weeks in the uterus.

Gestational age (GA):
the amount of time your baby has spent in your uterus. If he is 25 weeks gestational age he has spent 25 weeks growing in the uterus. This means he is about 15 weeks early, as most babies arrive between 38 and 41 weeks GA.

Extremely premature:
born having spent 24 to 28 weeks in the uterus.

Very premature:
born having spent 29 to 34 weeks in the uterus.

Moderately premature:
born having spent 35 to 37 weeks in the uterus.

Low birthweight baby:
a baby who weighs less than 5½ pounds (2500g) at birth. Most premature babies are also low birthweight. However, the two terms do not mean the same thing, because some babies can spend all 40 weeks in the uterus, but still be smaller than usual when they arrive. (See also **Birthweight** on page 14.)

Very low birthweight baby:
a baby born weighing less than 3⅓ pounds (1500g).

Extremely low birthweight baby:
a baby born weighing less than 2¼ pounds (1000g).

Term baby:
a baby who has spent the full amount of time developing in the uterus—between 38 and 41 weeks.

Viability limit:
how early a premature baby can be born and still live. Different hospitals have slightly different limits for the age at which they feel a premature baby can be helped. Although a very few babies have survived after being born at 22 weeks, viability limits usually fall somewhere between 23 and 25 weeks.

Nine out of ten premature babies survive and go home with their parents

Worrying though it is to see this tiny, vulnerable little being, your baby *will* change, develop, grow and mature—often more quickly than you imagined was possible when he began his life in such a fragile state.

"Such a tiny scrap of humanity, linked up to all those wires and dwarfed by machines. She didn't seem like a baby, more a half-human little animal, an essential component in a complicated life-support machine."

Pete, father of Emma, born at 27 weeks

Factors affecting what your baby can do

These include:

* Your baby's own particular personality and temperament

* His own special strengths and weaknesses

* How well he is and has been

* Any operations he has had

* Any medications he is receiving

* If and how he is being supported by technology—a baby on a ventilator can cope with far less than a baby receiving oxygen via a small nasal prong

* Whether he has recently had any tests (such as X-rays) or invasive procedures (such as regular clearing of his artificial breathing tube) that may have distressed or tired him

Birthweight

A baby's weight at birth also makes a difference to what he can do and with what he can cope. A baby born at, say, 32 weeks, might have the typical birthweight of a baby born much earlier—say, at 28 weeks. In this case birthweight can be a better guide to how he may cope than gestational age.

Low birthweight can (though does not always) mean that there were problems with development in the uterus, and your baby may show characteristics of or share problems with a more premature baby.

YOUR BABY'S PERSONAL COPING TIMETABLE

The information in this chapter is only a very general guide to what a premature baby looks like can do or cope with at a particular age. Babies are individuals from the moment they are born, no matter how early they arrive. What they can manage and when varies a great deal from baby to baby—even between those of the same gestational age—and depends on many different factors.

There are variations, too, within age groups. For instance, even though babies of 24 and 28 weeks are both considered "extremely premature," there can be an enormous difference between what an unwell premature baby of 25 weeks GA can do and cope with, and what a relatively well 28-week premature baby can manage.

IF YOUR BABY IS BORN AT 24 to 28 WEEKS

If your baby is 16 to 12 weeks early he is likely to weigh 1–3½ pounds (454–1600g). He will be about 10–13 inches (25–33cm) long, and spend most of the time—at least 80 percent of his day—trying to sleep.

How your baby may look

He will have a relatively large head—it is not yet in proportion with his body—and some downy hair on his face and body. This is called lanugo and is normal for the stage your baby had reached in your uterus. It appeared at 17–20 weeks and will disappear quite naturally at around the time your baby would have been born; hair on his back may rub off sooner, because he is lying on it.

He will probably seem very thin and fragile to you. As the fatty layer under the skin has not yet had time to build up, his skin will appear transparent: you can clearly see the delicate pattern of blood vessels threading their way across his body. His skin tone will usually be darkish red, at first, because his circulation may not be very good yet, and his blood may not contain enough oxygen. Your baby's skin may also look "waxy," but this effect will disappear as he matures. He may have some bruising on his skin, which is very sensitive to touch—even a monitor lead lying in the same place for a time can cause bruising. His skin is fragile and vulnerable to excessive handling.

Your baby's eyes may still be fused shut, like a newborn kitten's. All babies have their eyes shut from about ten weeks in utero to around week 26, when their eyes open naturally. When his eyes are shut, his eyeballs may bulge a little against their lids, and he may not yet have eyelashes. His ears are soft and flexible: if they are bent back they will not be able to spring back into position, as the cartilage in them has not yet formed firmly enough. He has the beginning delicate buds of fingernails and toenails, and perfectly smooth foot soles—there are no creases yet.

If your baby is a girl, her clitoris will seem quite prominent. Neither this, nor the protective folds of her labia will have grown. If your baby is a boy, his testes will

Ryan, born at 28 weeks

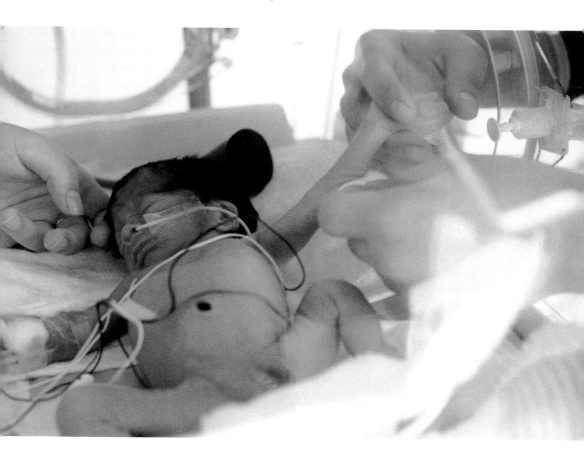

Why premature babies are thin

It is completely normal for premature babies to be thin, and the thinness is only temporary. They were born before they would have naturally started building up their layers of fat; in the uterus this begins at about 32–34 weeks. A premature baby who is healthy will usually begin to put on a little fat from around 32 weeks.

However, coping with the outside world before they are ready makes huge demands upon premature babies' systems. They need to use all their calories and energy for surviving and developing, and so have little left over to spend on getting fatter.

They are also under a great deal of stress, having to deal with things that they are not yet physically ready for—such as bright light, noise, touch, discomfort, pain or even breathing air. Just how much stress your baby may be under depends a great deal on how he is being looked after and protected, how well or unwell he is and how early he was born. But as he becomes stronger and more mature, he will be able to cope more easily.

When he no longer has to use all his energy just to survive, he will have some to spare for storing up in the form of fat padding and he will become chubbier.

not have descended and will still be tucked up inside his body. No nipples are visible on either girls or boys.

What your baby may be able to do

At this gestational age babies do not often have the energy to move much, but they may be quite active if they become agitated. Although his limbs are not strong, your baby may sometimes like to stretch, as he used to do in the uterus, and may occasionally bring his hand up to his mouth to try and suck his thumb or fingers, clamp his fingers into a fist or splay them open, or turn his head. If he can open his eyes for a few moments he may be able to see simple black and white patterns. He can hear sound; and he can certainly feel pain: all premature babies, no matter how early they were born, can feel pain.

Your baby can communicate using facial expressions and body language: yawning, hiccuping, arching his back, splaying his fingers (see page 86). He will probably be able to recognize voices—especially his mother's, perhaps also his father's, and maybe his brothers' and sisters' voices too.

From around week 28–29 onward, depending on how well or strong he is, your baby may be able to lick at breast milk expressed from your nipples, as a first step towards breastfeeding, and he may begin to learn to cup-feed (see page 117).

What your baby may not yet be able to do

He cannot lie curled up in the fetal position unless he is supported gently to do so (see page 93) but lies with his arms and legs sprawled out sideways. This is because his limbs do not yet have any active muscle tone. (This will start developing at around 34–36 weeks.) He won't be able to lift his head, and he may not be able to cry. More importantly, there are three vital things he probably cannot do for himself. He can't breathe all the time without help. Until they are around 32–36 weeks GA, premature babies' lungs do not produce enough surfactant—the substance that coats the inside of the lungs' airways and air sacs to help them stay open between breaths. Without enough surfactant, lungs collapse. This is why most premature babies will temporarily need some breathing support, ranging from a little extra oxygen to a ventilator (see pages 29–33).

Your baby also cannot keep himself warm. And he can't feed for himself. He will probably be able to suck, but premature babies of this age cannot coordinate their sucking, swallowing and breathing. This means he can't yet drink from your breast or a bottle without choking on the milk.

When your baby was inside you, he never had to worry about any of these things. Everything he needed you supplied, or did for him. He was warm in the shelter of your body. He did not need to breathe or eat because both food and oxygen came through the placenta and down through his lifeline, the umbilical cord. Now he is going to need some help for a while, until his systems are mature enough to take over.

For a description of the help your baby will be given, please see *What happens now?*, pages 22–81.

IF YOUR BABY IS BORN AT 29 TO 34 WEEKS

If your baby is born 11 to 6 weeks early, he will probably weigh between just over 2 to 5½ pounds (1000–2500g) and be about 12 to 14 inches (30–35cm) long.

How your baby may look

At 29 weeks he will not yet look like a smaller version of the traditional pink, chubby newborn. He will still have some growing, developing and, most of all, some weight-gaining to do. But a premature baby 34 weeks and older may well be starting to look much more like a newborn term baby.

However his head will not yet be in proportion with his body, and he will look thin. Some of his blood vessels may still show slightly through his skin; but these will become harder to see over the next few weeks, as he begins to build up a layer of fat. He will have soft downy hairs—called lanugo—on his face and body, and especially his back. This developed naturally in the uterus and will disappear over the next few weeks.

His small ears are floppy and do not yet spring back if they are folded down. This is because the cartilage that keeps ears in shape under pressure has not finished developing. The soles of his feet are relatively smooth, only having one or two creases on them. If your baby is a girl, her clitoris and inner labia will be fairly prominent

Wrinkle-free

Most medical books seem to say that premature babies have wrinkled skin. They don't—unless they are born very dehydrated, which is not common these days.

The myth dates back 30 years or more to the time when if a baby was born prematurely he was usually very dehydrated too, and this out-of-date information has stayed in the textbooks.

and visible because the outer folds of protective skin and soft tissue that form both labia have not yet finished growing. If your baby is a boy, you will see that his scrotum looks smoother than an older baby's. On both boys and girls, you can see the beginnings of nipples measuring $^1/_{16} - ^2/_{16}$ inches (1–2mm) across on their chests, though these are a fainter color than a term baby's.

What your baby may be able to do

He will be able to move his arms, legs, and body—sometimes quite vigorously—and his head from side to side. He may be able to grasp your finger firmly. He could probably suck on a pacifier if you gave him one and may be able to nuzzle at—and perhaps begin practice sucking on—his mother's nipple for comfort. If you express a few drops of milk and leave them on your nipple, your baby may be able to lick these off like a kitten—or even begin to try and breastfeed. Given the right support and help, he may be able to cup-feed from a special tiny, round-edged cup, licking and lapping at the milk (see page 116).

He may be able to turn his head toward the sound of your voice or another sound that draws his attention, and focus with interest on a face or picture about 10 inches (25cm) away (this is also the distance between his face and yours if you are holding him in your arms to feed him). He is likely to be able to recognize his parents' faces and/or voices—and perhaps his brothers' or sisters' too. He can feel pain, he can cry, and he can probably stay awake for short periods (beginning with a couple of minutes), alert and watchful, eyes wide open. He can communicate using facial expressions and body language and may be able to interact with you a little.

What your baby may not yet be able to do

He can't lie with his arms and legs curled close to his body in the fetal position, as you would expect a newborn baby to do, unless he is positioned in the right way and gently supported (see page 93). Instead, as he has so little muscle tone, your baby will lie with his arms and legs slightly akimbo, sprawled out to the sides. Nor can he yet hold his head up, if you pull him gently into a sitting position.

Ellen, born just seconds ago, after 34 weeks in the uterus

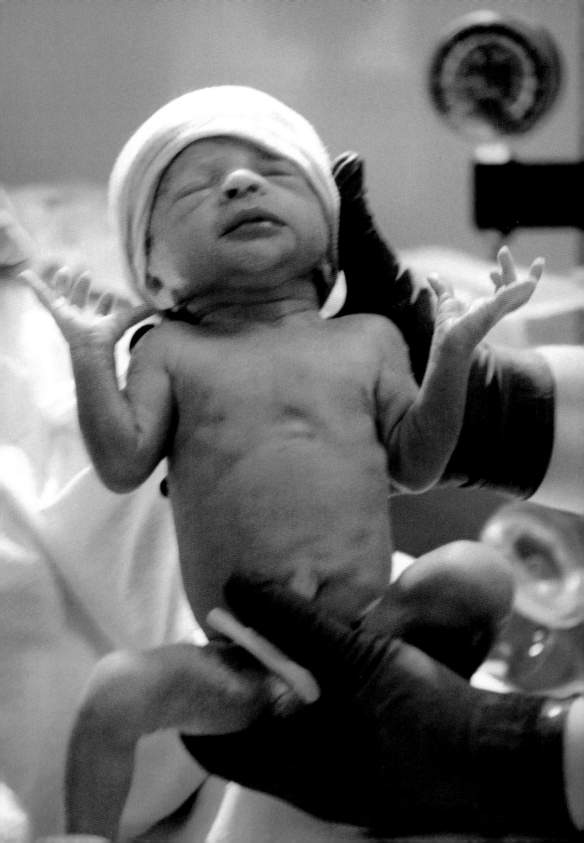

How can a 7½ pounds (3400g) baby be "premature"?

True, this is the average weight of a baby who has been in the uterus for 40 weeks. Yet it is not just your baby's actual weight that is important at this stage, but also how mature his body systems are. Each extra week in the uterus gives all these systems—breathing, digestion, temperature control, vision— vital extra time to develop.

A 7½ pounds (3400g), 35-week baby may be a good weight but still need a little extra help in these areas, even if it is only for a short while.

The help your baby needs

Premature babies may need a lot of extra care. Much of this, especially if they are very premature or unwell, is specialized medical care, and the next chapter details the many ways in which the hospital can help.

But babies have great need of their parents too, and there is an enormous amount that loving mothers and fathers can do to help, nurture and protect even the most fragile or tiny premature baby. To find out some more about this, please see *What can we do?* on pages 82–127.

Although he may be able to suck strongly, he is unlikely to be able to breast- or bottle-feed. Until they are around 34 weeks, premature babies find it difficult to manage to co-ordinate sucking, swallowing and breathing regularly and in the right order. This is why trying to drink milk by mouth may make them choke, so they need to take most of their food by tube, called a nasogastric, or NG, tube. Your baby will need extra help in keeping warm, and he will probably not be able to breathe without some help.

IF YOUR BABY IS BORN AT 35 TO 37 WEEKS

If your baby was born 5 to 3 weeks early, he will probably weigh anything from 3½–7½ pounds (1600–3400g) and be about 15–18 inches (38–45cm) long.

How your baby may look

At this gestational age, a premature baby will often look little different from a term baby. He may still have some of the soft downy hair, called lanugo, which formed naturally in the uterus, on his body, and perhaps on his face too, but this will soon disappear. He will probably be thinner than you would expect a term newborn baby to be. This is because the last few weeks in the uterus are spent putting on weight (see page 16).

His fingernails and toenails may not quite touch the ends of their digits. If your baby is a girl, her outer labia may not yet completely cover her inner labia, vaginal opening and clitoris. If he is a boy, both his testes may not have dropped into place. Sometimes only one will have done so, or either one or both testes will sometimes move back up into his body again. When this happens it is called having retractable testes.

What your baby may be able to do

If your baby is well and stable, he may now be beginning to cope with and do many more of the things that you might notice a newborn term baby doing. At around 37 weeks, his hands might be strong enough to hold tight to your fingers, as you slowly and gently pull him up. He may try to hold his head steady, and if you are holding him in a sitting position, he may try to bring his head up off his chest and hold it there for several seconds. Younger premature babies' movements tend to be weak and jerky, but your baby may now be able to move his arms and legs fairly strongly and smoothly and to bring his hands up to his mouth, sucking his fingers.

He will probably see almost as well as a term baby and enjoy looking at faces and patterns. He may try to follow your face with his eyes or turn his head to follow the sound of your voice, and turn to look up at you as you hold him close to your chest. He will probably recognize his mother's and father's voices, and perhaps any older brothers' or sisters' voices too. He may coo, or try to.

What your baby may not yet be able to do

If your baby is well, there may be little that a newborn term baby can do that he can't. However, even if he is able to breastfeed, bottle-feed or feed from a cup (see page 114) he may also need some temporary extra help in the form of tube-feeding. He may need help with breathing (perhaps just a little extra oxygen from time to time) and he will probably need extra heating to keep warm.

THE DEVELOPMENT OF THE BRAIN

There is a huge difference between what a 26- or 27-week GA premature baby can do and cope with, and what (if he is well) he will be able to manage just 6 short weeks later at 32–33 weeks. This is partly because the brain of a 26-week baby is very different from a 33-week baby's. The brain's surface, and therefore its capacity, develops very quickly between weeks 24 and 40.

Another important thing that happens in the 24–40 week period and helps a baby's brain to work more efficiently is that the system of ultra-fine "electrical wiring" that connects the brain and nerve cells together starts developing insulation. This process is called myelination. The signals passing from one brain cell to another are tiny electric charges and if they are to travel efficiently their pathways need to be insulated so they do not "leak." Myelin is the substance that develops to insulate the nerve fibers.

The surface of the brain

A 24-week-old premature baby's brain is smooth-surfaced, almost like a tennis ball. A 40-week-old term baby's looks more like a huge walnut. This is because from 24 weeks' gestation onward, the brain's surface has been folding itself into an intricate mass of ridges. And it is those ridges that are vital to learning and intelligence.

The brain's surface is the business part of the brain, the intelligent part. The surface cells are connected with the brain center, then the spine and body, by fibers that make up the bulk of the brain itself. The bigger a brain's surface area is, the more of those neurological connections it can make and so the more information it can process.

The folding, wrinkling process that goes on between 24 and 40 weeks is important because it increases a baby's brain's surface area enormously without taking up more room inside the skull. The end result is that the brain becomes far more powerful and efficient, so its owner can cope with more, do more and learn more.

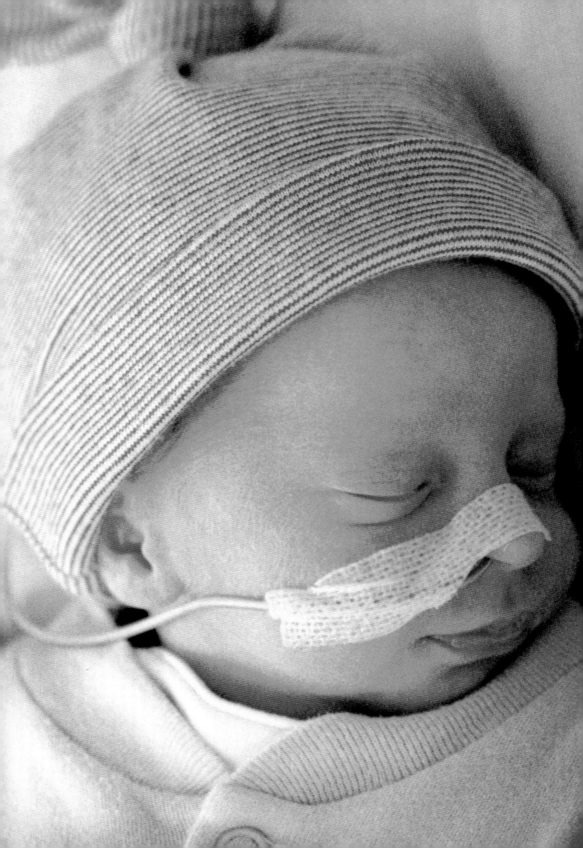

What happens now?

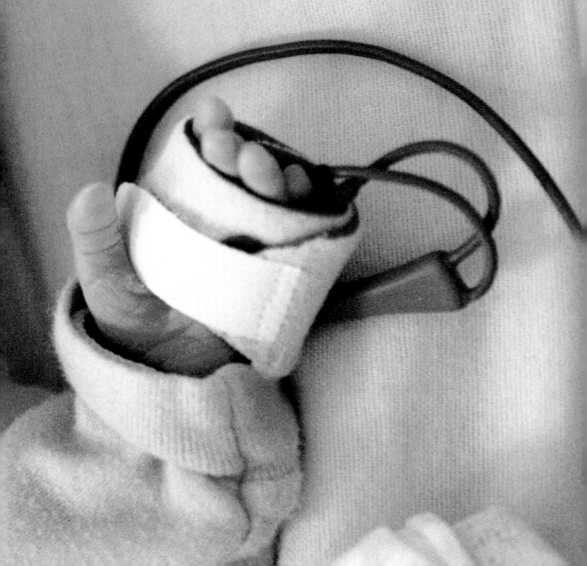

Names and abbreviations

★ **Neonatal care** is the specialist care of newborn (including premature) babies

★ **Intensive care** involves a major degree of advanced technological support and top-level staff expertise

★ **NICU:** Neonatal Intensive Care Unit, provides the most sophisticated level of care for babies, and is found at major hospitals and university centers

★ **Special Care Nursery** is for babies who have difficulties with feeding, breathing or infections but don't require the full care provided in the NICU

What does a Nurse Practitioner do?

An important complement to the medical doctor's role, nurse practitioners have received advance training that allows them to make assessments of a patient and design a treatment plan, including prescribing medications and ordering tests. They work as part of a team with doctors and specialists, NICU staff and the babies' parents to design the best possible program of care.

Your baby may now be in the unfamiliar world of the Neonatal Intensive Care Unit (NICU) and this chapter will try to introduce and explain the procedures and therapies she may experience and the machines, tubes and equipment surrounding her. It also looks at the possible reasons why your baby may need medical treatment—both minor medical problems that premature babies may have, and more serious medical conditions.

This chapter also looks at some of the many things that you, as your baby's mother and father, can do to help her, but for more detailed information, please see the chapter *What can we do?* on pages 82–127. Your love, care, watchfulness and protection are every bit as important to your baby's recovery as the skill of professional medical staff and the complex technology of the unit.

WHAT ARE ALL THOSE TUBES?

The first things that may strike you when you go into a neonatal unit are the heat, the bright lights and the number of machines that are in constant use. The initial impression for parents and visitors can be of a science fiction world whose complex equipment dwarfs the small babies being cared for there.

It can be both frightening and upsetting to see your baby lying in an incubator, attached to tubes and wires, surrounded by monitors that constantly flash and beep. Yet most parents say that they found that the more they knew about what the equipment was all for and how the different pieces of it were helping their baby, the less intimidating it became. If there is anything you are not sure about, the neonatal staff will be willing and happy to help you. Don't worry if you find you need to ask the same questions again and again. The nurses will expect this, and they will understand. They recognize that when someone is worried, tired and stressed (and you may be likely all three) it can be very difficult to remember even very basic information clearly the first time around. If you do not quite understand what a certain piece of equipment does, then many other parents before you—and many who will be at the unit after you—didn't or won't either. And as your baby's parents, if you need to know something, however small, then it *is* important.

GENERAL EQUIPMENT IN THE NICU

A premature baby may be born needing help with three very important and basic things: keeping warm, breathing and feeding. The equipment you see on a neonatal unit either will be helping your baby do any, or all, of these, or monitoring her to see how she is managing and checking whether she needs any additional support.

What follows is a general guide to the type of equipment you may see used to help your baby. Specific resources and procedures vary from hospital to hospital and you should never hesitate to ask for an explanation.

Incubator/Isolette

An incubator, or isolette, is basically a transparent plastic box on wheels. Its job is to keep your baby warm. Underneath it there is usually a cupboard for her things, such as diapers and any clothing. There are two main types of incubator:

Closed incubators have a lid, porthole windows and are double-glazed to keep in heat. A closed or lidded incubator also controls the amount of humidity (water) in the air surrounding your baby. This is important, as the hot, dry air of the NICU can dry out a baby's vulnerable skin. Small or sick premature babies may lose a good deal of water through their skin because they cannot control their own body temperature.

Open incubators have no lid or portholes, however, they do have an overhead heating unit and sometimes a specially heated mattress as well.

As your baby progresses and finds it easier to control her own body temperature, she will be able to move to an open crib.

Vital signs monitors

Vital signs is the term used for the indicators that show how well your baby's major body systems are working.

Levels of care

In some hospitals, your baby may be transferred from one "level" of care to another during her stay in the NICU. As some areas may have differences in how they define the levels of care, talk to your baby's caregivers if you have questions or concerns.

Level I provides:
★ monitoring of stable conditions
★ infant feeding, including breastfeeding
★ safe transfer to another level or hospital
★ emergency care if needed

Level II
In addition to Level I, provides:
★ care for newborns with birth weights of $3\frac{1}{2}$ pounds (1500g) or greater
★ continuing care of relatively stable, low birthweight babies
★ short-term or transport ventilation support
★ care for mild to moderate respiratory distress syndrome, suspected neonatal sepsis, hypoglycemia, and mild to moderate post-resuscitation problems

Level III
In addition to Level II, provides:
★ care for severe respiratory distress syndrome, sepsis, severe post-resuscitation problems, significant congenital cardiac and other diseases
★ severe complications and critical care
★ assisted ventilation on short- or long-term basis
★ specialist consultations
★ surgery and recovery care
★ transport care as needed

Vital signs include your baby's

⋆ Breathing rate

⋆ Heart rate (pulse)

⋆ Blood pressure

⋆ Body temperature

⋆ Blood gases: The amounts of oxygen and carbon dioxide in your baby's bloodstream and also how acidic or alkaline her blood is.

A Heart and respiration rates
B Oxygen saturation and heart rate
C Temperature monitors: isolette, baby
D Isolette/incubator

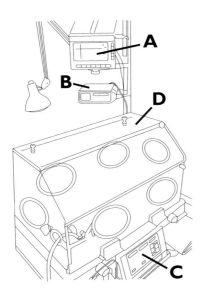

To check all or any of these vital signs, your baby may be attached to a monitoring system via small sensor pads with lead wires that are stuck to her chest. Several separate monitors can now be combined into a single machine that shows information for some, or all, of the vital signs on a TV-style screen. Which vital signs they will be monitoring depends on how well or unwell your baby is at the moment.

A **cardiorespiratory monitor** is a monitor that measures heart rate and breathing rate. An alarm goes off if either gets too far above or below the normal level.

A **pulse oximeter**, sometimes also called a **saturation monitor**, measures the amount of oxygen in a baby's blood using an infrared light sensor, which is usually attached to the baby's hand or foot. Monitoring oxygen is vital when a premature baby is sick. Too little or too much can be harmful, and may cause long-term health problems.

There are two main types of **blood pressure monitor**. Your baby's blood pressure can be measured either by wrapping a cuff (a mini version of the type used for adults) around her upper arm or by using a device attached to a line going into an artery. In either case the results are fed into a machine that automatically measures and then displays the pressure reading.

Ambient oxygen analyzer

This is a small device placed inside the incubator. It checks the amount of oxygen in the surrounding air.

IV line

IV stands for **intravenous**—the word comes from the Latin for "inside a vein." An IV line is a fine tube threaded into one of your baby's main veins. It may be in her arm, leg, scalp or umbilical cord. If she is very unwell or very premature, she can be fed through this tube. She can also be given extra fluids, extra nutrients or medications through her IV line. When an IV is required for a long time, a central catheter (or PICC line or long line) is inserted. This type of line lasts much longer than an IV line, which means fewer changes to the line and less discomfort for your baby.

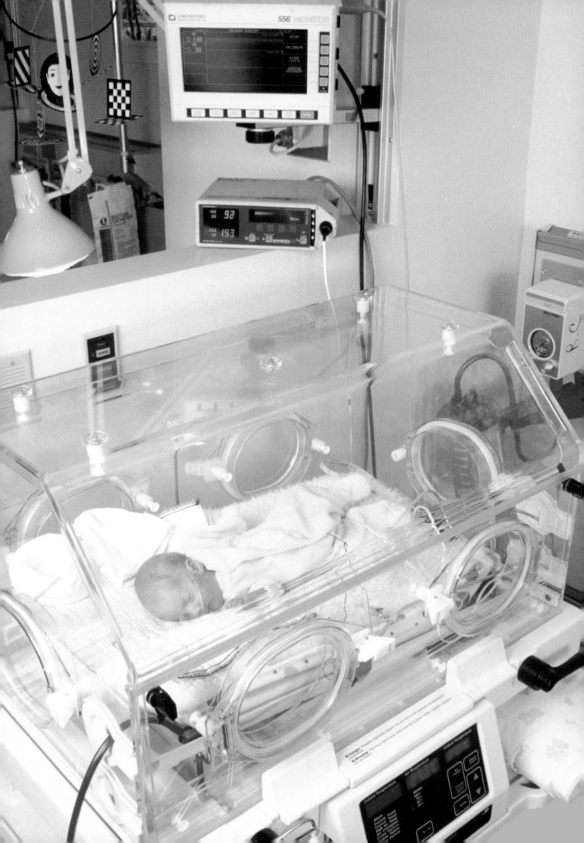

Alarming alarms

The sound of monitor alarms ringing is the backing track of every NICU. It never seems to stop (especially in the intensive care room) and it can be stressful for babies, staff and parents alike. Yet you may have seen that the nurses do not always seem to react.

In nearly every case this is not because they haven't noticed; they almost certainly have, but they know from experience that this is not an alarm that needs a medical response—this time.

This gets easier to cope with as you get to know and trust your baby's regular nurses and they get to know you and your baby. However, at first it can be very worrying and frustrating—and some parents remember it making them downright angry.

If you are worried, it may help to talk to the staff about your concerns and they should be able to explain how and when they think a medical response is appropriate—and when not to worry.

Nasogastric (NG) tube; orogastric (OG) tube; transpyloric tube

These are fine, flexible, plastic feeding tubes. A nasogastric tube is threaded through the baby's nose, an orogastric through her mouth, down her throat and into her stomach. A transpyloric tube goes directly to the baby's small intestine.

Umbilical catheter sensors

These fine plastic tubes are passed through an artery or vein in the baby's umbilicus (belly button). They can be used for giving her fluids, nutrients and medications, or for taking blood samples. Some NICUs also attach to these lines special machines that can measure your baby's blood pressure and/or the level of oxygen in her bloodstream.

Phototherapy unit

This is a lamp unit that shines bright light—not ultraviolet light—onto a baby's naked skin. It is used to help treat jaundice, usually successfully (see page 47).

Biliblanket

This is a special mat made of soft fiber-optic tubes that emit bright light, which the baby lies on. Biliblankets are used as another way of giving a jaundiced baby phototherapy treatment.

Apnea alarm

If a baby stops breathing for more than 10–20 seconds, she is having an apnea attack (see page 34). This is a common problem for premature babies, though most have stopped having these attacks before they leave hospital.

In the meantime, your baby may need either to wear an apnea alarm around her tummy, or lie on a special flat alarm pad placed underneath her mattress. The alarm will sound if she stops breathing for a certain (brief) period of time. Very occasionally, a baby may go home with one of these alarms (see page 172).

SPECIAL EQUIPMENT TO HELP WITH BREATHING

Many premature babies have problems with their lungs and need some extra help with their breathing. Some may only need a little help for a few days. Others may need high-tech support from a ventilator for many weeks, even, occasionally, months.

Extra oxygen, headboxes and oxygen masks

This equipment is used for babies who can breathe without help but need some extra oxygen. Air with extra oxygen added to it can be delivered straight into a covered incubator. It may also be piped into a special clear Plexiglass box called a **headbox** which rests over the baby's

Archie is being fed through a nasogastric tube, and a nasal cannula is helping him to breathe.

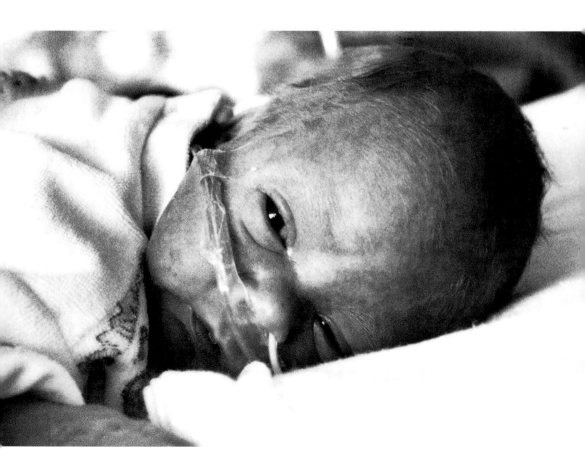

29

head, or it is delivered via an **oxygen mask**. The box and the mask can be used in an open incubator.

Nasal cannula

This is a way of delivering extra oxygen to your baby through her nose using two tiny tubes (one in each nostril). These are attached to slim, flexible plastic piping that goes back across each cheek, behind the baby's ears and then along to the source of oxygen.

Oxygen analyzer

When a baby is receiving extra oxygen, the level is always measured very carefully by an analyzer. This is usually a small plastic sensor placed near the baby's face or somewhere along the oxygen route.

Humidifier

If your baby needs long-term oxygen therapy, the air and oxygen mixture is often passed through a humidifier first. This moistens and warms the gases: something that a term baby's nose does naturally.

CPAP

This stands for **continuous positive airway pressure**. It usually involves a mixture of air and extra oxygen being blown through two small tubes placed in your baby's nostrils and down into her lungs to help keep the air sacs open after each breath. It keeps them slightly inflated—as they are in an adult or a term baby—even after exhaling, to ensure that they do not collapse, and prevents the inner surfaces from sticking together. The result is that the baby does not have to make such an effort to draw each breath. CPAP can also be given via an endotracheal tube (see below).

Ventilator

This is a machine that helps a baby breathe or, if necessary, can take over the process completely. A mixture of air and extra oxygen is gently blown or pushed down a pipe called an **endotracheal tube (ET)**. The tube leads from her mouth or nose, down her throat and into her airways. Some babies may need ventilator support for just a day or two, others may need it for many weeks or even months.

Being attached to a nasogastric tube doesn't stop Ellen from enjoying a cuddle. (She's doing her best to pull the tube out, though.)

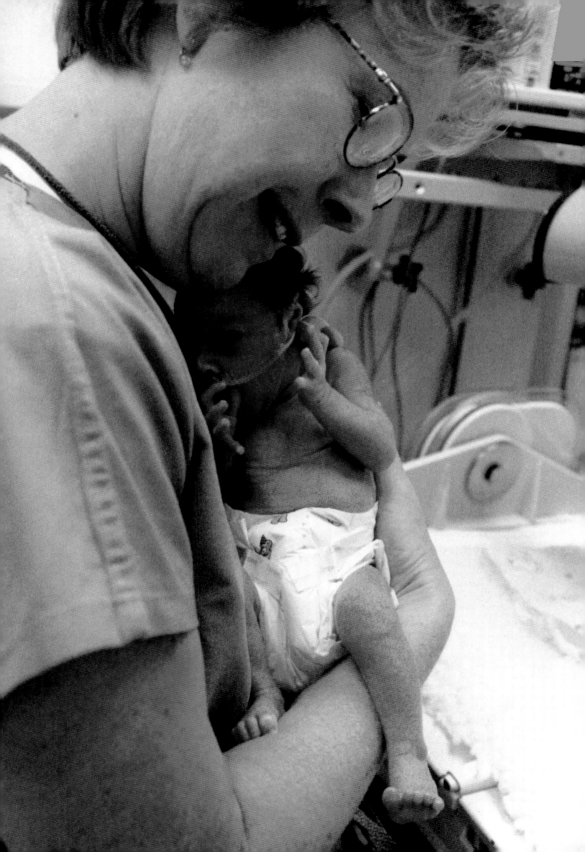

There are several different sorts of ventilator. A large regional neonatal unit may offer them all, though a small NICU may only have one or two. The type of ventilator a baby will have depends on the sorts of problems she is experiencing. If she needs a special ventilator that the unit does not have, she may well be transferred to a hospital that does.

There are two main types of ventilator:

A **positive pressure ventilator** pushes a mixture of air and extra oxygen under carefully controlled pressure through a soft ET. This air flows down into the baby's lungs and helps them to expand normally as she breathes in. Breathing out also follows naturally when the machine stops puffing the air, allowing the baby's chest to fall again. The ventilator puffs down 20–40 "breaths" per minute, on average. A baby will stay on the ventilator until her lungs

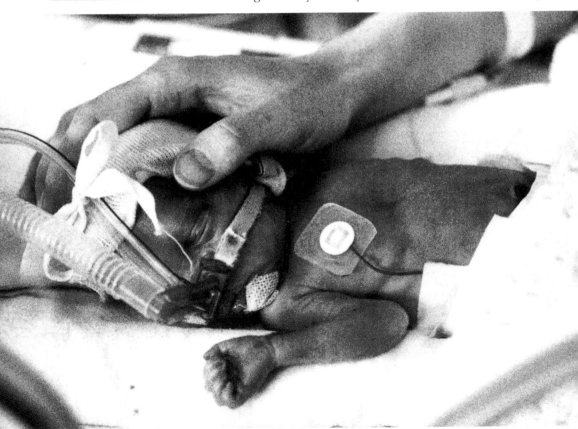

CPAP helps George breathe. He is being fed through an orogastric tube, and his vital signs are constantly monitored via the sensor pads stuck to his chest.

are mature enough to cope alone, or have healed from whatever damage they have suffered. The weaning-off-the-ventilator process is careful and gradual.

Some positive pressure ventilators are highly sophisticated. For babies who cannot breathe without help at all, they will do all the necessary work. Other babies can cope with taking at least some breaths themselves, and the machine can allow them to do this in between ventilator breaths. There are also some types of positive pressure ventilator that babies can trigger themselves. These machines wait for a baby to begin to take a breath herself, then gently blow in some extra air mixture at the same time, to give a helping hand.

An **oscillatory ventilator** or **high-frequency ventilator** still uses an ET to deliver the air mixture into the baby's lungs. But it delivers smaller puffs of air and extra oxygen at a much faster rate: instead of being blown down, the gas is "vibrated" down. A baby supported by this type of machine does not look as if she is breathing, as such, at all. Her chest doesn't rise and fall, but shakes with vibrations. This type of ventilator is much gentler on the lungs.

ORDINARY MEDICAL PROBLEMS

This part of the book should be used only as a reference section to dip into when you want to know something about a specific problem. It should not be read from start to finish right off the top. It is only about the *possible* health problems your baby may face—it is not a list of all the illnesses she will definitely have. Many are either completely normal things for premature babies to experience temporarily, or they are common conditions that can be treated easily and effectively.

It is far more likely that your baby will develop, say, two or three of the difficulties mentioned in this section, and then only for a short time. Most of these will either sort themselves out as your child matures, or they can be treated by the NICU staff without any lasting ill effects.

Serious problems

The more premature a baby is, the more difficulties she may experience and the more serious these may be; the less premature she is, the fewer and less serious the difficulties are likely to be.

For less usual but more severe problems, please see the section starting on page 57.

"Every time she stopped breathing for even a few seconds, it was like my own heart stopped. We tried to be cool about it, like some of the other parents who would just sigh, and rub their baby's feet to get things going again. But we just never could get quite used to it."

Steven, father of Chloe, born at 34 weeks

However frequently your baby pauses for breath, you can expect a big improvement when she reaches 31–33 weeks (gestational age).

Because your baby has been born ahead of her time, her body is not yet ready to adapt to life outside the shelter of your uterus and she may have some difficulties at first. Here are some of the most common problems a premature baby may need to deal with, together with information about all the things that both the NICU and you, as your baby's parents, can do to help your child.

Many of the most common health problems for a premature baby, such as difficulty keeping warm, apnea and cyanosis (from low oxygen levels), happen because her nervous system has not yet finished maturing, so it cannot yet keep many of the body functions stable and even. The more premature a baby is, the more of a problem she will have with this, though babies can mature surprisingly fast if they are basically well and properly cared for. There are enormous differences between what a 28-week premature baby can handle and what a 34-weeker can manage.

APNEA (BREATHING PAUSES)

Premature babies often stop breathing for a few moments. As a matter of fact, so do many newborn term babies. If the pauses only last from 5–10 seconds before they re-start by themselves, the condition is called periodic breathing. This periodic breathing is a harmless and perfectly normal thing for a new baby to do, and because it doesn't cause a baby any problems it doesn't need any treatment. However, if your baby's breathing pauses are longer, say nearer 10–20 seconds long, this is known as **apnea**. These breathing pauses may cause her heartbeat to slow (this is called bradycardia, see page 36) and her skin to become pale, mottled or bluish. African-American babies tend to show they are short of oxygen by having darker lips, a darker area around their noses and a darker than usual color on their tongues.

Most premature babies have apnea. Some studies have found that they spend as much as 12 percent of their breathing time pausing. The more premature your baby is, the more likely she is to have apnea, and the more mature a baby is at birth, the less likely. Apnea is usually caused by the immaturity of your baby's nervous system, lungs and airways; though in some cases there may be something blocking her breathing tube—for instance, her tongue may relax back into her throat while she is asleep because it does not yet have enough muscle tone to keep itself in its proper position.

Apnea tends to start, if it is going to, within a day or two of a premature baby's birth. It only lasts until her breathing and central nervous systems mature, which may take anything from a few days to several weeks. If your baby is on a ventilator, this hides signs of apnea, which may then appear when she begins breathing on her own.

What staff may do to help

Often no one will need to do anything, as your baby will usually start breathing again on her own. If she doesn't breathe within 20 seconds or so, a nurse will help her to start breathing again by gently rubbing or stroking her side or foot. If this doesn't work, staff will try giving extra oxygen. They may do so by gently blowing a stream of oxygen near your baby's face; or by "bagging"—carefully pumping extra oxygen into your baby's lungs using a small oxygen bag, plus a mask.

If a premature baby has frequent apnea spells, staff will monitor her carefully so that they can act fast if any trouble develops, or she may have extra help with her breathing for a while.

Checking and helping your baby's breathing

The medical staff may attach her to a pulse oximeter (see page 26) that tracks the amount of oxygen in her blood. Alternatively—or perhaps as well—she may be connected to a cardiorespiratory monitor (see page 26) to keep a check on her heartbeat and breathing rate. Both machines have alarms that go off if your baby's oxygen levels, heartbeat or breathing rate drop even slightly below a certain level. Or she may just be attached to an apnea alarm (see page 28).

Your baby could also be given some continuous help. This may be in the form of nasal CPAP (see page 30) or

Medication-watch

If your baby is being given theophylline or caffeine, keep an eye on her behavior. Staff will be monitoring her too, by maintaining a careful record of the levels of theophylline in her bloodstream (though they tend not to check caffeine levels).

Both types of drug are very useful for apnea, and caffeine is useful for bradycardia, but their side-effects can include restlessness and irritability, and they may occasionally make a premature baby vomit or send her heart rate up.

If any of these reactions occur, ask your baby's caregivers whether perhaps another approach that doesn't have these side-effects could be used instead.

If a premature baby is on medication that is making her unsettled, this will affect her rest and sleep, which are vital to her growth and recovery.

medicines such as theophylline or caffeine to stimulate the central nervous system (see page 35).

What parents can do

Although it can be really alarming to see your baby's breathing pause, try not to panic. It's completely natural to react strongly if you see your baby stop breathing for even a few seconds—those few seconds can seem like a very long time—but premature babies can take far longer breathing pauses than can adults without any apparent ill effects. If possible, try not to focus only on the breathing pauses or, in isolation, on the readings on any monitor she may be connected to. Instead, look at your baby closely to see how well or comfortable she seems and how healthy her color is, because these are things that are just as important.

If the breathing pauses are too long, you need not feel you have to stand by and do nothing. Try rubbing your baby's feet gently but firmly. This will usually stimulate her to begin breathing normally again. If it does not work within 20 seconds, call a nurse to help you.

Outlook

The likely outcome for your baby is excellent. Premature babies grow out of apnea as their breathing systems mature. Many parents worry that there might be a link between apnea and the likelihood of SIDS (see page 171). However, a recent (1996) study about this suggests that although premature babies are more vulnerable to SIDS than babies born at term, this is because they are more likely to have a range of health problems—not because they have experienced and then grown out of apnea spells.

BRADYCARDIA (SLOWING HEARTBEAT)

The hearts of most premature babies beat roughly 120 to 160 times a minute (this is about twice as fast as yours). If your baby's heartbeat slows down to less than 100 beats a minute, this is known as **bradycardia**. This temporary slowing of the heart is most usually caused by an apnea spell but, occasionally, bradycardia may be the effect of a heart problem.

What staff may do to help

The staff's response to bradycardia will generally be similar to their treatment of apnea (see page 35). They will rub your baby's foot gently but firmly, and if that doesn't have the desired effect, they may give her some extra oxygen. They may also keep a check on her by attaching her to a cardiorespiratory monitor (see page 26), and if they think some continuous help is necessary they may give her caffeine medication. However, in many instances they may do nothing, except watch the baby carefully. The slowing might not be too far from the normal range and she may recover without any help.

What parents can do

Rub your baby's foot gently but firmly. If this doesn't seem to help, or if you are worried about her because she seems

Heart and respiration monitors help NICU staff keep a close watch.

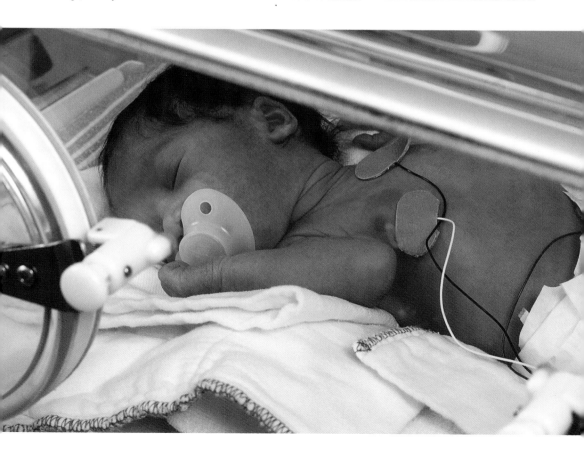

distressed or doesn't look well, ask a nurse to come over to check on her.

Outlook

The likely outcome for your baby is excellent. So long as the bradycardia spells are not caused by a heart problem, she will grow out of them as her nervous system and breathing mechanisms mature.

CYANOSIS (TEMPORARILY BLUISH SKIN)

A baby's skin often has a blue tinge in the first few hours after she has been born, especially if she is cold. No matter how warm delivery rooms may be they are up to 20°F (11°C) colder than it was inside you.

If your baby has slightly bluish fingers and toes, this is likely to be what doctors call **peripheral cyanosis**, which is caused by the immaturity of her circulation control system. This can lead to congestion (sluggish circulation), but is not usually a problem.

However, if your baby has a bluish color around her mouth, a bluish tongue or lips or an all-over bluish-pink or "dusky" skin tone, she may well have the more serious **central cyanosis**. On darker-skinned or African-American babies the bluish tinge is not so easy to see, though experienced neonatal staff can spot it. Often a color change can be seen inside a darker-skinned baby's mouth or on her tongue, or a paler area around her nose and mouth.

Central cyanosis needs to be dealt with urgently because it means that your baby is not getting enough oxygen. There can be many reasons for this, including the possibilities that: her heart may not be pumping oxygen-rich blood around her body fast or effectively enough; she may not be breathing effectively; she may have an infection; or she may be cold.

What staff may do to help

If apnea seems to be the cause of the trouble, they will rub your baby's feet gently to re-stimulate her breathing. If the breathing problems are more serious, they may give her some extra oxygen or further assist her breathing. If she is too cold, they will give her extra warmth and make sure she keeps warm.

What parents can do

Rub your baby's feet gently if she is having an apnea spell, and see if she is warm enough by feeling the back of her neck or her body; it is not a good idea to check her body temperature by feeling her hands and feet—these may give a wrong impression because, as her circulation is not mature yet, they are very often chillier than the rest of her body. If you are still worried, ask a nurse to come and check your baby.

Outlook

Unless the cyanosis is due to a serious health problem—for example an abnormality in the way your baby's heart has developed or a lung condition such as BPD (see page 61)—she will grow out of it naturally as her breathing system and heart mature.

FRAGILE SKIN

A premature baby's skin is very delicate. It has a thinner, far less fatty bottom layer than a term baby's, and the top layer is thin and fragile, so it doesn't protect the middle growing layer well and it's not so securely attached. Your baby's skin will be thinner than a term baby's; it will tend to be dry, to absorb anything put on it too readily and to be easily damaged—even the gentle removal of a bandage can cause a minor wound. Therefore it can easily get infected. The earlier a baby is born, the more delicate her skin will be.

What staff may do to help

There are many things the staff can do to minimize damage to your baby's fragile skin. They may use special medical tape for securing things like IV lines and dressings and will put soft barriers between your baby's skin and the sticky part of the tape. For example, dabbing any sticky tape that is going to be laid against her skin lightly against cotton coats the tape in a light protective fluff; this makes it less likely to remove any delicate skin when the tape is taken off again. When sticky tape needs to be taken off, the nurses can use warm water to loosen it first, before pulling

Skin

Skin is actually made up of three layers.

1 *Epidermis*: the protective top layer

2 *Dermis*: the middle or growing layer

3 *Subcutaneous tissue*: the fatty bottom layer which helps keep out the cold.

Together the layers act as a barrier against the outside world.

Flaky skin

Your baby's skin is likely to go through a quite normal dry and flaky stage as it matures: try to resist the powerful temptation to put on creams to moisten it—it won't help in the long run. If you are worried that your baby is not comfortable, talk to a senior member of staff to see what they can suggest.

Weight loss

The smaller or more premature babies are when they are born, or the more unwell they are, the more weight they will lose at first. Full-term babies lose 5–10 percent of their weight just after they are born, but premature babies lose nearer to 10–15 percent.

it away gently. Your baby's caregivers will use only warm water—no soaps—for washing her, and not put creams, lotions or other substances on her skin unless absolutely necessary, because they can be absorbed too easily.

Because the air in the NICU is so hot and dry, it takes vital moisture from your baby's skin. The drier the skin is, the more likely it is to tear or crack, so staff may add water vapor to the baby's environment in the incubator to keep the air around her more humid. They will always try to touch your baby as gently as possible and may wrap her in a soft material, such as a sheepskin blanket, for extra protection.

What parents can do

Try to make sure that anyone who touches and handles your baby does so very gently and washes their hands before and afterward. Check that her nurses use some sort of effective barrier between her skin and any sticky medical tape securing IV lines. If they are not doing this, and especially if you notice a sore place on your baby's skin where tape has removed a small area of it, talk about it with a member of staff whom you like and trust.

Outlook

Your baby's skin may be immature but it is developing quickly. Within a few weeks the top layer will be less dry and flaky and almost as securely attached and strong as any newborn term baby's.

LOSING WEIGHT / NOT GAINING WEIGHT

It's normal for babies to lose weight just after they are born, whether they have spent their full quota of 38–41 weeks in the uterus, or arrived early. There are usually two (generally harmless) reasons for this. First, your baby is getting rid of the extra water and salt in her system that she doesn't need any more; she had a lot of both when she was still in the uterus. Secondly, term and later-born, more mature premature babies being breastfed will for the first few days be receiving colostrum, or pre-milk. This marvelous fluid is rich in minerals, vitamins and antibodies to fight infection, but not high in the calories that help a baby put on weight.

Even when your baby begins to gain weight, she may not put it on steadily at first. Premature babies need more calories because everything is more of an effort for them, and they may be taking in less food than they need. If they are distressed or uncomfortable, they may spend energy (calories) trying to cope with this or moving frantically. Very premature babies have a higher metabolic rate too, and this is another reason why they may need more food than they are able to take in.

Premature babies have tiny stomachs and can only take a little nourishment at a time. Provided they are well, however, their stomachs can usually hold enough food for their needs if they are fed at least every two to four hours. (Some babies may need to be fed a tiny amount continuously via a drip or a tube.) Problems arise if something, say repeated vomiting, is stopping your baby from taking in or retaining the food she needs. If she has a gut problem, this will also prevent her from absorbing enough nutrients from the milk she has taken in.

What the staff may do to help

The nursing staff will set up a careful feeding regimen—and measure your baby's weight and growth regularly—daily if she is unstable or unwell, or every few days if she seems to be growing steadily. They will make very sure she is getting enough fluids. Just how much your baby needs is calculated exactly, even down to the number of drops needed per minute for some very small babies.

Your baby is likely to be losing water through her thin, fragile skin, so caregivers will try to make up for this by adding extra humidity (moisture) to the air. They will also make sure she stays warm, so that she does not waste calories trying to generate her own central heating. If that vital energy has to be spent on keeping warm it cannot be used for growing. The caregivers should generally also be trying to keep your baby calm and comfortable. Stress and restlessness also use up calories your baby needs to spend on growing.

What parents can do

If you spend a lot of time watching your baby carefully you will be in the best position to judge whether she is

"Every day we'd ask: 'Has she gained?' and would worry if she hadn't, or even worse, had lost weight. A good day for us was her putting weight on, a bad day was when she lost some …"

Martine and John, mother and father of Zoe, who was born at 29 weeks

41

Premature babies get cold very easily for three main reasons:

1 They are born before they have laid down much fat under their skin, so do not have much natural heat insulation.

2 When older babies and adults are cold they generate their own extra heat by shivering. Newborn babies cannot shiver, and for emergency heat supplies they burn up a special sort of fat, called brown fat, instead. Premature babies have very little of that, and none at all if they are less than 30 weeks old.

3 The bigger a body's surface area is relative to its weight, the faster heat is lost from the body and the more easily it gets cold. All babies have a much bigger surface area relative to their weight than adults and the ratio for premature babies is even higher than for term babies, so they lose heat fastest.

A nurse takes Nina's temperature, using an electronic thermometer. The baby's hat is a vital piece of equipment that prevents her from losing heat through her head.

comfortable. Anything you can do that reassures her, comforts her or helps keep her calm can be really valuable: the more relaxed and at ease your baby is, the more calories she can save for growing and putting on weight. There are many things that you, as your baby's parents, can do to help make your child calmer and more comfortable, even if she is very unwell; there are some ideas and suggestions in the next chapter, *What can we do?*

Try not to be discouraged if your baby loses weight for a couple of days, even if she had been putting it on steadily before. This is normal. Every baby is unique, and they all have their own special patterns for putting weight on— maybe gaining for a few days, staying still for a couple, then losing weight again for a couple. You can get a clearer idea of how your baby is doing if you average out her weight gain over a week. It also a good idea to take a long look at the baby herself: that will tell you more than just a weight chart every time. How does she seem to you? Is her color OK, does she seem fairly peaceful and comfortable? This can mean more than any temporary fall in weight.

Outlook

Your baby will grow bigger and stronger steadily as her body systems become more mature, though this may happen more slowly if she has been very unwell or was especially fragile to begin with.

KEEPING WARM

All premature babies need some extra help with keeping warm. But of all the things they need, this is the one that NICUs can deal with most easily. Neonatal care units are very warm places anyway (which parents and staff know to their cost, as they are often uncomfortably hot for adults).

Unit staff will also use everything from incubators, overhead crib warmers and pre-warmed oxygen to blankets, baby bonnets and bubble wrap to help make sure your baby does not become chilly. Even so, both you and they need to keep a constant lookout for signs that your baby is cold (see page 162). Being cold can make a baby ill,

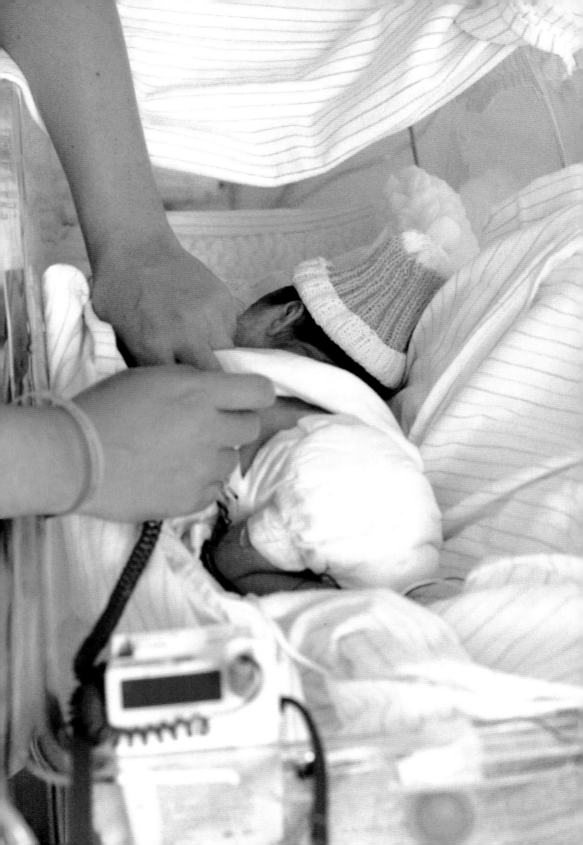

One very good way to keep your baby warm is by kangaroo care (see page 105). This is skin-to-skin contact with your baby, with her snuggled up on your chest or between your breasts, down inside your shirt. Your own body heat is a natural means of keeping a baby, especially a premature baby, warm and it can be a lovely way for both parents to soothe and feel close to their baby.

because it may cause breathing problems, low blood sugar levels and weight loss.

Also, when premature babies get cold they have to use up some of the energy they get from food to make heat—and this is energy they need to spend on growing. Most early-born babies have their work cut out to take in just enough food to grow, so wasting energy on keeping warm slows down their growth and weight gain.

What staff may do to help

Everyday precautions against your baby getting cold include warming up everything before it's used on or for her: hands, incubator, blankets, sheets, clothing, mattress, washing water, drying towels, incubator or crib—even warming up any extra oxygen the baby is given so it doesn't arrive in a chilly stream. Staff may put a warmed blanket on any cold surfaces your baby is placed on, such as weighing scales or X-ray plates, even if it's only for a moment. They should protect her from drafts, keeping her away from doors in constant use, from windows and from potentially chilly outside walls.

Staff will monitor your baby's temperature regularly and if there is a problem, they will use incubators, heated mattresses and overhead warmers, sometimes putting side-guards on the warming unit or stretching plastic wrap over the sides and end of it. They will probably give her a soft cotton bonnet to wear all the time, as everyone, babies and adults alike, loses a lot of heat via the head. And they will probably not wash your baby very much because even when using warm water and a warm towel, some water will still evaporate off your baby's skin as she is being dried and this cools her body down fast.

What parents can do

See if your baby's nurses are taking the precautions outlined above—if they are not, ask if you can talk to them about the ways they can help keep a baby warm and which they might recommend for your child. When you hold your baby in your arms or on your lap, make sure she has a hat or bonnet on, and use a soft blanket to wrap around her.

If her temperature tends to fall easily at the moment, try to resist the understandable urge to wash her. It's very natural for parents to want to wash their child: this is part of the usual baby care mothers and fathers instinctively do for a newborn, and the wish to do so can be very strong. You may feel you'd especially like to wash your baby or have the nurses do so if she has little flakes of matter on her skin, such as dried blood or the remains of the soft waxy substance called vernix that covered her skin when she was in your uterus. Yet these will not cause an infection or hurt her in any way and in the interests of keeping your baby warm it may be best to leave washing for a while. Talk to the nurses about this if it is bothering you—perhaps just her face could be dabbed gently?

Outlook

As your baby grows stronger and bigger, she will be able to keep herself warm more easily.

JAUNDICE

Jaundice shows itself as a yellowish tinge to your baby's skin and/or gums and to the whites of her eyes. In darker-skinned or African-American babies, yellowing of the whites of the eyes is often the only visible sign (Caucasian babies may look as if they have a slight suntan). The yellow tinge is caused by a pigment called bilirubin, which is produced when old red blood cells are broken down. If the liver cannot remove bilirubin quickly enough, it builds up in the blood and gets deposited in the fatty layer just below the skin, showing through as a yellowish color.

Jaundice itself is not a disease (although it can sometimes be a sign of some conditions, such as an under-performing liver), and it is very common in all newborn babies, full-term and premature alike. This is because all babies are born with extra red blood cells they no longer need outside the uterus and, perhaps more importantly, it usually takes three to four days for even a newborn term baby's liver to start working efficiently enough to remove bilirubin from the blood. It is normal for a premature baby's liver to take five to ten days to remove this yellow

Up to 8 out of every 10 premature babies develop what doctors and nurses call physiological (or "newborn") jaundice—but so do up to 6 in every 10 term babies.

material, but it can take far longer. The more prematurely the baby was born, the longer it may take.

Generally harmless and straightforward to treat, jaundice is still a condition that no one can afford to ignore as it can sometimes be a sign that the liver is not working properly. If it becomes severe, it can cause further problems, including possible brain damage. Even at its mildest jaundice may make your baby drowsy, slow to feed and listless, and since premature babies tend not to have much energy and find feeding difficult at first, this can make things worse.

What staff may do to help

Physiological or "newborn" jaundice often clears spontaneously after a few days, but in any case staff will keep a close watch on your baby's bilirubin levels using

An eye mask shields the baby's eyes from the bright lights used to treat jaundice, while mom's touch offers comfort.

Photo: Glamour International/First Light.ca

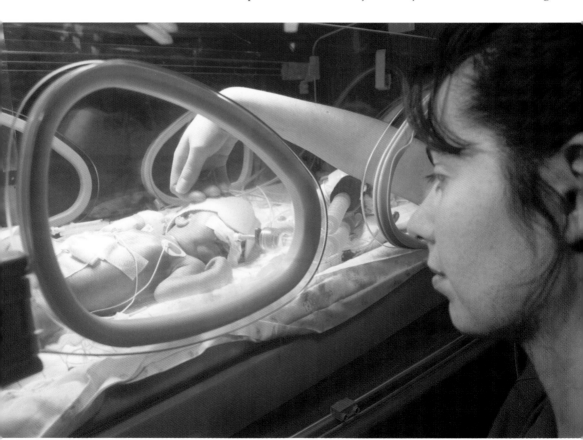

simple blood tests. If they think she needs treatment to clear the jaundice, they will use phototherapy.

Phototherapy (treatment with bright lights) works by making the bilirubin molecules change their shape, into one that is easier for the body to get rid of. Your baby will lie in her incubator, naked but for eye shields, under warm, bright lights that are left on 24 hours a day—in effect "sunbathing" her jaundice away, though the lights are not damaging UV rays. Sometimes a fiber-optic light blanket called a Biliblanket (see page 28) is used instead.

While she is having phototherapy treatment, your baby may develop a light rash, but this will vanish after treatment stops. She may also be sleepier than she usually is and have either runnier bowel movements than normal or none at all. It is important that the staff give her extra fluids because, like sunbathing, phototherapy can be dehydrating. Premature babies can lose nearly twice as much fluid as usual when they are having light treatment, so this is very important.

Phototherapy works so well that it is usually the only treatment a baby will need. However, if your baby is too severely jaundiced for phototherapy to be effective she may be given a blood transfusion. This can take several hours and will be carried out by a doctor who will not even need to move your baby from her bed. Sometimes a baby will need a series of exchange transfusions, spaced over a couple of weeks.

If the jaundice carries on for a long time, the doctors will check out possible causes including metabolic problems, thyroid disease, blockages in the baby's bile ducts, or liver infection. Depending on the problem, treatment may be medication (metabolic and thyroid problems), surgery (blockages) or antibiotics (infections).

What parents can do

It is very helpful if you can be there to calm your baby when she has her regular heel-prick blood tests to check bilirubin levels. Ask the medical staff if they can use any of the methods outlined on the right to minimize the pain. Premature babies find it especially hard to calm themselves

Blood tests—minimizing the pain

If the nurses warm your baby's foot in their hands (or if you do this for your baby yourself) before trying to take a blood sample, this can make it easier to take the sample, and her foot will be less likely to need uncomfortable squeezing.

Some units use local anesthetic creams—either lignocaine or amethocaine—put on the skin up to half an hour before the prick to help deaden the area. Most specialists will not use the better-known EMLA cream (which can be given to term babies and toddlers or older children), as it gets absorbed too readily into a premature baby's fragile skin.

47

down again after becoming distressed but if you are there to comfort and soothe your baby she will settle down again far more quickly. Ask the caregivers to advise you when tests are to be carried out so you can be there to comfort your baby.

During phototherapy, you can still take your baby out from under the lights to hold, feed and cuddle her—or even to give her a bit of kangaroo care—if she is medically stable. There is no reason why the 24-hour light treatment cannot be interrupted for 30–60 minutes at a time, at least once a day, for this. You can also talk to or stroke your baby while she is under the lights (but perhaps not both, as this can be too much for premature babies). Let her know you are still there for her.

Usually babies undergoing phototherapy can carry on feeding as before. Although breast milk can sometimes make the jaundice last longer, possibly because of the hormones it contains, you shouldn't be discouraged from feeding her your breast milk if you've been able to make and/or express some—it's still the best food she could possibly have.

Outlook

Unless the jaundice has been very severe, it will clear up quickly with no harmful effects.

ANEMIA

If your baby has anemia it means that her blood does not have enough red blood cells. Red blood cells carry vital oxygen around the body; if there aren't enough of them, your baby's heart will have to pump harder to make the most of what oxygen is available. This makes her tired, and she may also have to breathe faster to get more oxygen. All babies, whether they are full term or premature, become slightly anemic after they are born. In healthy term babies, this sorts itself out naturally within their first three or four months. Premature babies are more likely to need treatment, for two reasons.

First, a premature baby has missed the last weeks in the uterus. Babies get most of the iron they need from their

The smallest premature babies may only have 1½ fluid ounces (40ml) of blood, compared with around 8 pints (5 liters) for the average adult woman. Because of the regular tests they need, a premature baby can lose the equivalent of what to you would be 1 pint (1 liter) of blood every week.

mothers in the last 12 weeks of pregnancy. Iron is essential for making healthy red blood cells, and important for preventing anemia. If your baby was born early she would have missed out on some, or perhaps all, of this.

Second, the problem is compounded by the fact that your baby has so many blood tests. These are mostly routine ones, taken day after day: tests for blood gases, blood glucose, hemoglobin count, electrolytes... The nurses take as little as possible each time, and hospital labs try to devise tests that only need tiny amounts of blood, but it still adds up. The amount of blood taken for each test varies from as much as 5ml when they are first admitted to the NICU—this can be one-eighth of a premature baby's entire supply—to as little as 0.2ml for a regular blood gases check. Most tests need nearer to 1ml each, and they may in some cases have to be carried out two or three times every day.

There are some other possible causes too, but these are much less common than the two above. They include a mother and her baby having incompatible blood types or the mother bleeding before her baby was born, perhaps because her placenta was positioned over the cervix (placenta previa). There are also some infections that can trigger red blood cell breakdown.

If the anemia comes on suddenly, your baby will be very obviously ill. She will look pale, have clammy skin and a fast pulse, and she will need extra oxygen. Tests can show that she has a low level of red blood cells and hemoglobin (the substance that does the actual oxygen-carrying, and makes blood red-colored). If the anemia comes on slowly you may notice that she gradually becomes less active (how easy it is to spot this depends on how active she was before) and that she looks pale and floppy. If she is feeding from a bottle or your breast she will seem to find this harder and more tiring. She may gain weight only slowly, or not at all, and she may also need extra oxygen.

Anemia is not that much of a problem for a premature baby if it's mild and is effectively monitored and treated.

Can I be my baby's blood donor?

Some parents are very keen to give blood for any transfusions their baby may need. In many countries using blood donated by parents is routine. The best thing is to ask your baby's nurse what the procedures are to request this for your baby.

However, if it is not spotted and becomes severe, it can cause serious breathing and heart problems.

What staff may do to help

Your baby's doctors or nurse practitioners will do a blood test to check if her hemoglobin or red blood cell counts are low. Sometimes they don't need to do anything further except keep a sharp eye on the condition, so long as it is not making the baby unwell, because anemia often rights itself in time.

If your baby's anemia needs further investigation, they may do some more tests to check the size and shape of her red blood cells, look for any signs that the cells are being destroyed and check for any risk of bleeding in the baby

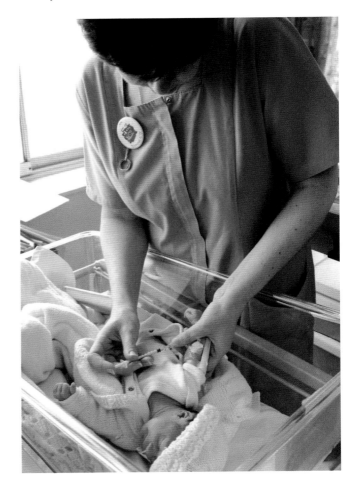

A nurse administering medication through an IV line.

herself. NICU staff may well give your baby extra iron and folic acid too, but she will only need the folic acid until she reaches the day she should have been born; the iron can be stopped as soon as she is growing well and eating some solid food. (Iron may give your baby diarrhea or constipation—and because it tastes unpleasant it needs to be disguised in her food or milk.)

Some NICUs will give an anemic baby weekly injections of a hormone called erythropietin, a chemical that the kidneys usually produce naturally, though this is not a universal practice. (Speak with the nurse if you have questions about this.) Premature babies' kidneys make this too, but not enough of it. Erythropietin stimulates the bone marrow to make more red blood cells. If your baby is very unwell with anemia, or if she is not yet too ill but her anemia is gradually getting worse, she will be given a blood transfusion.

What parents can do

If you spend time just sitting and watching your baby, you will get to know what is normal behavior for her and what is not, so you will notice any signs of anemia or, if it has already been spotted, whether it is getting worse or better. Tell the nurses what you notice.

Outlook

Unless the anemia was the result of some kind of a massive, uncontrolled blood loss, your baby will make a complete recovery, with no lasting ill effects.

SEPSIS (INFECTION)

Premature babies are especially vulnerable to infection. A premature baby's immune system has not yet had time to develop fully and grow strong, and because she was born early she has missed out on some of the infection-fighting antibodies she would have got from her mother, over the last three months of pregnancy. In addition, the necessary and life-saving treatments premature babies need to grow and survive often invade the baby's small body by breaking the skin barrier. Injections, heel-prick tests, an IV line into her arm or leg or sometimes her scalp, vital equipment

Sepsis

Sepsis is the medical term for an infection—of any sort.

The most common infection is probably septicemia (a general infection of the blood, see over) followed by pneumonia, gastrointestinal infections, skin infections around the umbilical cord area, urinary tract infections and meningitis.

There is information about some of these more severe infections on pages 57–81.

How can my baby get infected in the hospital?

Your baby might have caught the infection before she was born. If you had the infection while you were pregnant, the infectious agent (bacteria, a virus or a fungus) might have crossed the placenta and entered your baby's body.

Some infections can be passed to a baby as she is being born, while she is traveling down the birth canal. And, if the waters break 24–48 hours before labor proper begins, because the barrier of the amniotic sac is torn, an infection can find its way through the tear in the membrane to reach the unborn baby.

However, your baby may well have caught the infection in hospital, from staff, visitors, equipment or other babies on the unit. Despite everyone's best efforts, even NICUs can never be completely sterile places.

such as catheters or breathing or feeding tubes placed partially inside her body—all of these offer a possible way in for germs. Your baby may need several of these treatments and procedures at once, for days or even weeks. And each one carries a risk of infection with it.

How infections arise

An infection develops when a germ (bacteria, a fungus or a virus) gate-crashes its way into a part of the body that can't fight it off. There it multiplies, causing pain or making you unwell. For instance, if you cut your finger and bacteria get in through the break in the skin, they will breed there, causing the area to swell, redden and hurt. But your body's immune system can usually contain the germs. This means the infection usually stays in your finger and doesn't spread to the rest of your body. An infection for a premature baby however usually entails more than a sore finger, because a premature baby's immune system is not yet strong enough to keep the germs trapped in the area where they first came in. So, often the infection spreads, causing a general infection in the blood. This is a condition called **septicemia**, which means "infection of the blood;" it is sometimes called blood poisoning. If septicemia is not spotted and treated early enough, it can make a premature baby very ill.

How to tell if your baby has an infection

It is sometimes hard to tell whether a premature baby has an infection. The signs may only be subtle and gradual, or they can be dramatic and show themselves fast. It depends on how severe the infection is, and what the cause is.

You might think that one of the most obvious signs would be a high temperature, as it is for a term baby, a child or an adult. It isn't. If anything a premature baby is more likely to be slightly chilly—hence some of the signs you see might be those of central cyanosis (see page 38), such as a bluish tinge to your baby's skin if she is Caucasian, or to the mucous membranes in her mouth if she is darker-skinned; or she may just have pale or mottled skin and chilly hands and feet.

She may have trouble with her breathing, perhaps breathing very quickly (this is known as tachypnea), or with her chest sinking right in when she breathes, or even with long pauses between breaths. You may have difficulty with her feeding and she may have diarrhea or vomiting. She may have seizures (see page 77), or be irritable, jittery and jumpy, or perhaps be listless and just generally seem unwell. There may be noticeable signs such as jaundice or spots, a rash, even a discharge perhaps from her eyes, nose or other infected area.

However, *all* these signs may be symptoms of other things too, and your baby may not have an infection at all.

Gentle touch calms and soothes this baby girl. The mittens prevent her from inadvertently scratching herself—as well as removing the monitor leads or feeding tube.

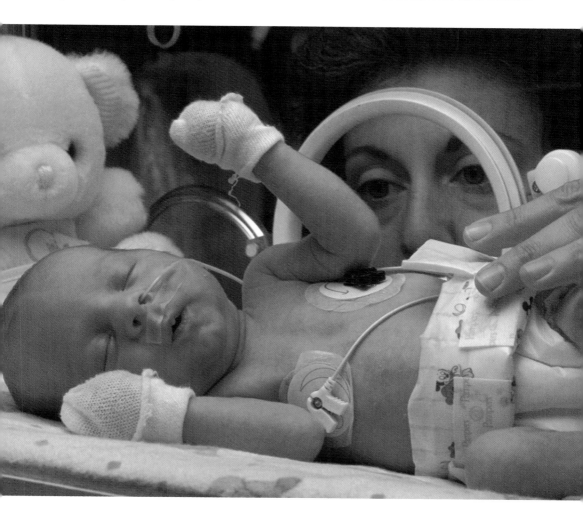

Cough and cold caution

If you are the mother of a premature baby and have a mild cold, it is very unlikely that you would need to stay away from your own child unless she is either very unwell or extremely fragile and the staff advise it for a day or so. The good that you can do just being there beside her far outweighs the risk of her catching your germs. Newborn babies seldom seem to catch infections from their mothers anyway. However, anyone else— including father, brothers and sisters, grandparents—should stay away from the baby if they have even the mildest sniff of a cold or other infection.

Even when a baby is sick and in a closed incubator, a loving parent can get very close.

Tests

If the staff suspect an infection, they will take samples of your baby's blood, urine and perhaps spinal fluid too. These are given to the hospital lab to see if they can grow (culture) any bacteria, viruses or fungi from the samples. They may also test samples of mucus from your baby's nose or chest, or take a swab from any wound site to check for infections there. They may take X-rays of her chest or abdomen or make an ultrasound scan of her abdomen.

What staff may do to help

To prevent infections, staff will wash their hands thoroughly when they first come into the NICU and then should always thoroughly wash their hands again after dealing with one baby and before going on to touch another. They should also follow strict hygiene rules for all equipment, and always be on the lookout for any sign of infection.

If an infection has already started, or doctors strongly suspect one, they will give your baby antibiotics immediately, without waiting for any test results. Premature babies are not yet strong and can become very ill very quickly, so doctors will usually give your baby broad-spectrum antibiotics (a catch-all antibiotic that tackles most general infections) right away, as lab results may take several days to come through. When they do get the results of the tests, they may change your baby's medication to give her one that targets her particular infection more specifically or more effectively.

What parents can do

Like the staff, you will be following strict hygiene rules, such as washing your hands thoroughly with medicinal soap and hot water before and after you handle your baby. Ask all your baby's visitors to do the same.

If your baby is ill with an infection, stay by her as much as you can, as your presence and love will help her tremendously. There are also many specific practical ways you can comfort your baby even if she is very sick or fragile, some without even touching her at all. (Please see the next chapter, *What can we do?*)

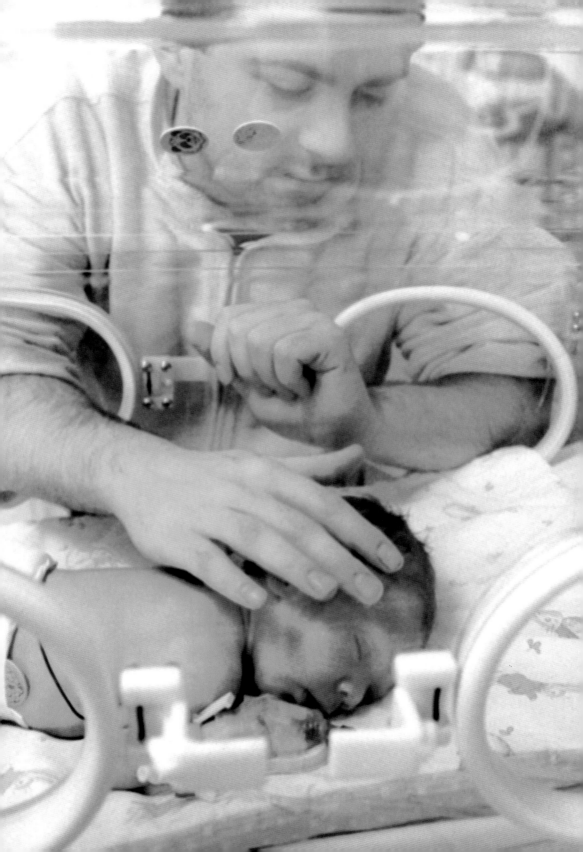

Shock

Shock is the medical term for the collapse of the blood circulation system.

Its effects include inadequate blood flow, not enough oxygen reaching the tissues and waste products not being removed properly from the blood. Symptoms include cold, sweaty, pale skin; a fast, weak pulse; a dry mouth; irregular breathing; and dilated pupils.

Shock can occur when a premature baby develops sepsis, suddenly loses a great deal of blood or has heart problems or even a severe allergic reaction.

When it comes to telling whether your baby has an infection, you have a special advantage because, as her mother or father, you will probably know more about her than any of the staff, and you may instinctively know when your child is not herself. Neonatologists say that often parents will notice that something is wrong a good 24 hours before doctors are convinced. Typically, they say, parents usually notice first, then the nurses, who know the babies better than the doctors do, and lastly the doctors, because they are able to spend the least time with any individual baby and know them least well.

This is especially likely if you have been able to spend time sitting beside her and just watching her, because you will have had the chance to absorb a good deal about her own special signs and body language (see page 86). You will also probably have been getting an increasingly good idea about what is normal for your baby, and what isn't. If she just does not seem quite right to you but you cannot put your finger on precisely why this is, tell a nurse you like and trust and with whom you have a good rapport.

Outlook

Antibiotics usually clear up most bacterial infections completely and antifungal medications can be effective. There are only a few antiviral drugs, so for many viral infections NICUs must rely on "supportive care" to increase the baby's ability to fight off the infection—this means giving the baby as much extra help as she needs with breathing, keeping her warm and comfortable, giving her extra fluids to avoid dehydration and so on (they will give this supportive care to any sick baby, but will redouble their efforts for a baby with a viral infection).

Mild to moderate infections tend to leave no trace. But if an infection is severe it may cause other problems. In the short term, some release toxins (poisonous waste matter) into the blood; in addition to making your baby feel unwell, this can stop the blood clotting properly and so cause bleeding problems. If the infection interferes with a baby's blood pressure or the way her heart works, she may also go into shock (see left). It may also have altered the balance of certain vital substances, such as sodium, potassium, calcium or glucose, in the baby's blood. This can have harmful effects: for example, too little or too much potassium can affect the way the heart works.

There are plenty of treatments for these complications. These include administering clotting agents, helping the baby's blood pressure to stay stable with extra fluids and medications, keeping her warm and well fed, giving her extra oxygen, using a ventilator, giving mild sedation to slow down the amount of oxygen she is using up and reducing her fluid intake or adding certain chemicals and substances to it.

Some severe infections may cause longer-term damage that takes time to heal properly. These infections are discussed in the next section.

SERIOUS MEDICAL PROBLEMS

Your premature baby may only have a few fairly minor health problems which are easily treated and then graduate relatively smoothly and quickly from her stay in the NICU to going home with you. But some babies can have serious difficulties, punctuated by repeated setbacks. This section takes a look at some more serious disorders and at the many things that can be done about them.

This section may at first look a bit alarming—pages and pages giving details of one problem after another. However, it is not really meant to be read all the way through. Instead, you might like to use it by just turning to the relevant section if you'd like to find out more about a specific condition that your baby has, or one that she looks as if she may develop.

What you will find here is a basic factual account of each problem, its treatment options and likely outcome, which you can use as a secure base for building up your own special knowledge about your baby's particular needs, using both the information from the neonatal staff about your baby's health and progress, and your own powerful instincts as her parents. This may make it is easier to ask the doctors and nurses specific, informed questions that will give you the true picture of how your baby is doing.

"There is no such thing as a bad question, or a question asked too often."

Debbie Askin, Neonatal Nurse Practitioner, St. Boniface General Hospital, Winnipeg

WHAT PARENTS CAN DO

As the parents of a sick or very fragile premature baby you can be desperately anxious and may feel fearful and helpless. Many mothers and fathers whose premature babies have been ill however, say, that it helped them greatly to find out all they could about their baby's condition and treatment. It may help to write down all the questions you would like to ask on a small notepad you can carry with you easily—and their answers too. Ask a lot of questions, and ask them as many times as you need to. Experienced medical staff will expect this and understand.

Protecting and supporting your baby

Never discount the value of your presence to your baby's progress.

Even if you cannot physically pick her up and cuddle her, there is a great deal that you as your baby's mother or father can do to comfort and protect your child when she

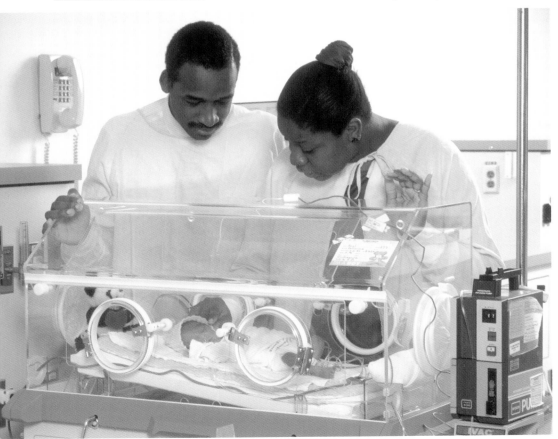

is very unwell, or to soothe her before and after an invasive investigation or operation. You also know or will come to know far more about your own baby than anyone else. If you would like some ideas or suggestions about supporting your baby, see the next chapter, *What can we do?*

RESPIRATORY DISTRESS SYNDROME (RDS)
Sometimes called HYALINE MEMBRANE DISEASE, or IDIOPATHIC RDS (IRDS)

Respiratory Distress Syndrome may develop if a baby's lungs are not mature enough or big enough to work properly, or if the baby is not making enough surfactant, the substance that usually coats the insides of the tiny air sacs in the lungs and stops them from collapsing inward. Without surfactant these air sacs (called alveoli)—which make up the lungs—sag inward between breaths, making it harder for the baby to take the next breath. A baby with RDS may have a real struggle drawing air down into her lungs. This can be exhausting, and it also means she is not getting enough oxygen. Fluid may then seep into the sacs, which makes it even more difficult for them to stay inflated with air.

The more prematurely a baby is born, the more likely she is to have this condition and the more severe it can be. About half of the babies born at less than 30 weeks have RDS. In premature babies, making enough surfactant for their breathing to ease can be a slow process: the earlier a baby arrives, the slower the surfactant build-up, and the more help she will initially need with her breathing.

Symptoms

Neonatal staff can diagnose RDS just by looking at a baby and how she is breathing. Some babies show clear signs of RDS right from birth. The most obvious of these are: the pulling in of the skin and muscles between or just below the ribs (retractions) as the baby tries to breathe; grunting, or panting as she breathes; and the flaring of her nostrils as she tries harder to draw in air. She may also have bluish, dark red or mottled skin, or bluish membranes inside her mouth, showing that she's not getting enough oxygen, and apnea spells.

Serious breathing problems

Of all the potentially serious problems a premature baby may have, breathing problems are the likeliest. Your baby's doctors will probably use respiratory distress syndrome as an umbrella term for breathing difficulties which have not been going on for long. If problems persist (become chronic) they tend to be referred to as chronic lung disease or bronchopulmonary dysplasia (see page 61).

"Giving surfactant treatment automatically to all appropriate babies would save 1,400 premature babies' lives every year."

Richard Cooke, Professor of Neonatal Medicine at Liverpool Women's Hospital

Treatment

There is a very wide variation in how badly a premature baby may be affected by RDS. She may have it so mildly that the condition can safely be left to sort itself out without treatment. However, even if it is mild, the neonatal staff will still monitor her carefully to make sure all is well. If she has RDS more severely, a single dose of surfactant treatment (see below) is often enough to deal with it. But, sometimes, a baby's breathing difficulties are more acute and she will need breathing support (perhaps from CPAP or a mechanical ventilator; see page 30) and she may also need repeated surfactant treatments before she is better.

Surfactant treatment

Artificial surfactant fluid is given via a tube placed in the baby's windpipe. The thick liquid then drains gently down into her lungs. This is quite a specialized procedure and is most successful when it is carried out at a major NICU where the staff are highly experienced in administering this particular treatment. As a back-up, a baby may also be given some extra air and oxygen using CPAP or a ventilator.

The policy now in most major NICUs is to give surfactant automatically to babies with RDS because if this is done the chances are they will not need any ventilation treatment at all. Babies can also be given surfactant at birth if they just look as if they might develop RDS, rather than waiting until they have already developed it.

Outlook

Mild cases often sort themselves out; less mild cases may only need a single dose of surfactant and be fine after that. Even severe cases have a good likely outcome, especially if surfactant treatment and additional breathing support are given promptly and correctly to the babies who need it.

However, if RDS becomes severe or is not treated properly, it can cause serious long-term breathing problems such as BPD, eye damage (retinopathy of prematurity), IVH, a heart problem called patent ductus arteriosus, or necrotizing enterocolitis (for these problems, see the entries that appear below).

BRONCHOPULMONARY DYSPLASIA (BPD)
CHRONIC LUNG DISEASE (CLD)

These are two different names for what is basically the same chronic (long-term) lung disorder. BPD/CLD is most often seen in premature babies who have had particular difficulty breathing and therefore have needed the help of artificial ventilator machines for several weeks to help them survive, although it also occurs in babies whose lungs have been damaged, for example by a pulmonary hemorrhage.

Your baby being on a ventilator does not necessarily mean she will develop BPD. However, if these machines need to be used for long, they can damage a premature baby's fragile lungs, causing BPD.

BPD can be very frustrating because it is something of a vicious circle. Very small or premature babies' lungs are often not mature enough or strong enough to cope with breathing air without some major help and they may need time on a ventilator. Yet the force at which ventilators push air into the windpipe can damage the baby's fragile lungs, which will then find it even harder to work properly. This means a baby may possibly become dependent on the machine for her breathing—while her lungs continue to be damaged by the very device that is keeping her alive.

Symptoms

The damage to the lung itself involves scar tissue formation, which causes small areas of the lung to collapse altogether, while other areas trap air and balloon out. This is why, in X-rays, the lungs of a premature baby with BPD look bubbly.

BPD also affects the breathing tubes—the windpipe and tiny bronchioles in the lungs—causing them to produce too much mucus, which can clog them. It also causes twitchy, asthma-like spasms that interfere with breathing; in fact, if anyone in the parents' families has asthma, this can also be a risk factor for a premature baby developing BPD.

Ventilators

Since they were first used in the early 1970s, ventilators have made an enormous difference to the care of very sick premature babies, saving the lives of many thousands who would otherwise have died. Babies do not usually need a ventilator machine for long and most can be gradually weaned off it in less than a week.

Pneumothorax

This is the medical term for air in the tissues surrounding the lung and and its effects include acute respiratory distress. A pneumothorax occurs when air "leaks" into the chest cavity causing the lung to collapse. To treat it, a tube is inserted into your baby's chest and X-rays are taken to make sure it is in the right place. The chest tube usually stays in a few days and is removed once your baby's condition has improved.

Treatment

Chest X-rays will confirm whether or not your baby has BPD. She will need to be on a ventilator until she can breathe without it, but if possible staff will use an oscillatory or high-frequency ventilator (see page 33) as these are usually the gentlest on the lungs. Unfortunately, not all hospitals have these, as they are very expensive. The NICU will wean your baby off the ventilator very gradually. After this she may be supported with CPAP (see page 30) before finally graduating to breathing on her own.

Staff will also make sure your baby is getting extra calories, because she will be using a lot of energy, fighting to breathe if the machine allows her to take her own breaths in between ventilator "breaths," and generally handling the stress of being constantly on a ventilator. She cannot breast- or bottle-feed, so she will have extra nourishment fed though a nasal tube or catheter. Staff may possibly give your baby some gentle chest physiotherapy, too. This can include delicately tapping her chest area with a finger or a tiny cup.

Medical staff may also, depending on your baby's needs, give her medications. They could give her stimulants such as theophylline or caffeine to stimulate her breathing, or sedatives and anti-anxiety drugs if she is becoming distressed by being on a ventilator. Diuretics may occasionally be used to help stop fluid from collecting in her lungs. If she is in pain the staff may give her painkillers: either a short-acting drug such as fentanyl, or a longer-acting powerful one from the morphine family.

Coping with babies in distress

Babies can become distressed or agitated while they are on ventilators. It cannot be comfortable having a tube in your windpipe, often having no choice but to breathe with the rhythm of a machine rather than your own natural rhythm. They may also be in pain, or lying uncomfortably. Premature babies who have BPD can be especially sensitive to light, noise and being handled, and become exhausted very easily as the strain of being on a ventilator rapidly uses up all of the very little amounts of energy they have.

Ten weeks after his birth he is still scarcely bigger than his father's hand. He needs a nasal cannula to help him breathe and he is being fed through a nasogastric tube. There is a long way to go. But he is out of the incubator and off the ventilator and father and son can find comfort in a cuddle.

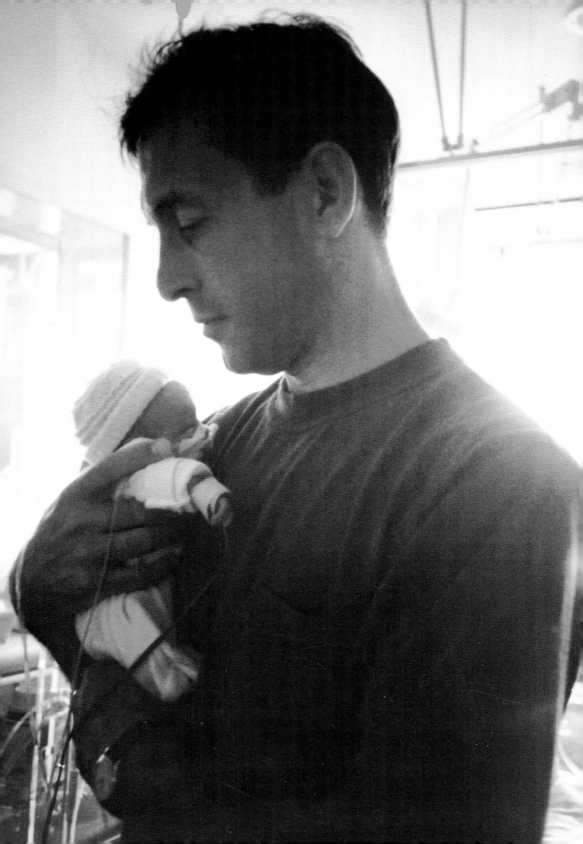

Can my baby become addicted to painkillers?

Premature babies may well become temporarily physically dependent on drugs such as painkillers, sedatives or anti-anxiety medication if they have needed them for a while. Medical staff will therefore make very sure that any drugs like this will be tapered off slowly, never ever stopped suddenly.

If your baby has needed to have this type of medication for a couple of weeks or more, talk to her nurses about whether physical dependence might be a problem for her. If they feel this is possible, ask them how she is going to be weaned off her medication once the time is right.

According to Dr. Kathleen VandenBerg, of the Children's Hospital in Oakland, California, they may also have the sense of fear that can come from being "air hungry" or unsure about their breathing capacity.

One answer to this agitation and distress is sedatives. These will calm a baby down; but if she is in pain, these drugs may also give the baby's caregivers the impression that she is content, when she is not. In fact one study (see *References*) suggests that sedative drugs may actually make babies more sensitive to pain, not less. Anti-anxiety drugs, too, can make a baby more peaceful but may mask pain.

However, babies who have BPD are not easy to comfort. They can be hard to bond with or relate to as they are so often stressed, agitated and exhausted. This can be difficult for parents trying to get close and give love to their babies. Your baby may tend to squirm and arch herself away if you try to hold her, or simply turn away or shut her eyes because, in her distress, she cannot even cope with her parents' faces trying to make loving contact with her. This can be really disheartening, enough to make even the sanest and most competent, calm and loving mother or father feel helpless and inadequate.

If your baby has BPD and is behaving in this way, try to remember that it is not you she is rejecting. It's more likely that she is finding the situation she is in too much to cope with, and she is trying to handle it in the only way she can—perhaps by trying to shut everything out or pulling away from any other form of stimulation, like a cuddle, your voice or your face. But she does need you badly. She needs to feel your presence beside her and she needs your love, your help, your support and protection in ways that she *can* cope with. See the chapter *What can we do?* for some ideas that may help.

Outlook

A baby or child with BPD who has the right constant care will get better, even though she may be anything from three months to six years old before her breathing is totally problem-free. She will need to be weaned away from the ventilator, or from extra oxygen help, slowly and gradually; for a while she may still need extra oxygen

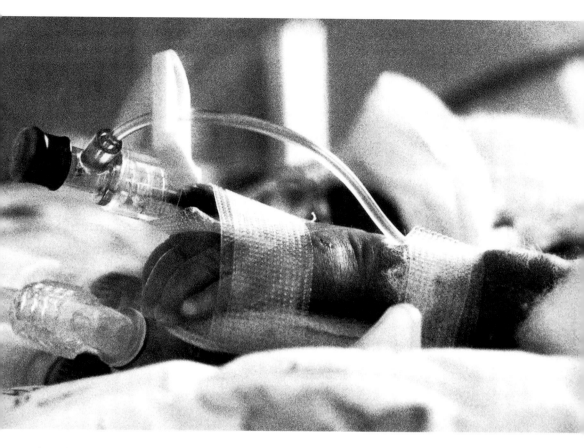

while feeding from your breast or a bottle. A very few babies who are otherwise well will go home with oxygen equipment and continue their therapy at home to help their lungs carry on strengthening and healing. (See the section on caring for babies who need extra oxygen for a while at home in *Time to go home*, page 169.)

An IV line provides a vital channel for medication or fluids. Bound to the baby's arm, a splint helps to hold the line secure.

PATENT DUCTUS ARTERIOSUS (PDA)

When a baby is still developing in the uterus, she has a short passageway or duct called the *ductus arteriosus* (DA) linking two of the big blood vessels leaving the heart. In an unborn baby, the DA links the main artery supplying the body, called the aorta, with another big artery, the pulmonary artery, which takes blood from the heart to the lungs. This passageway is meant to close up soon after she is born. But in some newborns, usually babies born

PDA is one of the most common heart problems for premature babies. Around one in five of premature babies who weigh less than 3 pounds 5 ounces (1500g) when they are born has PDA.

prematurely, this small connecting passageway may stay open; or it may close, and then open back up again. When this happens, the condition is called **patent** (open) **ductus arteriosus**.

While this duct stays open babies do get enough oxygen, but their lungs may get too much blood to cope with. This can cause some serious side-effects, especially if the baby is very premature, such as fluid gathering in her lungs or, if her lungs stop working properly, becoming (and then possibly remaining) dependent on an artificial ventilator. The good news is that PDA often sorts itself out with time, and it may be so mild that it causes your baby little or no problem at all.

However, if a baby is very unwell or fragile she will not be able to afford to wait for the condition to correct itself and she will need treatment for the PDA before it starts causing complications.

Symptoms

PDA is usually diagnosed from the sound of your baby's heart heard through an ordinary stethoscope; the doctor may be able to hear the "continuous murmur" sound that it makes. Other signs include the baby's blood-pressure reading, any trouble she may be having with her breathing or if she has an unusually powerful pulse which may be seen or felt anywhere—in the groin, wrist or top of the foot, for example.

PDA can be confirmed by an X-ray of the heart or a Doppler ultrasound scan (a type of scan that can show movement) to check how the blood flows throughout the heart.

Treatment

The treatment the doctors decide on will depend on how big the PDA opening is, and how much difficulty it is causing. If it is not too serious, they will try reducing the amount of fluids in your baby's body. Usually a diuretic medication (one that will make her urinate out excess fluid) will be tried first and this is often successful.

If the PDA is more serious, however, they may decide to use a medication called indomethacin. If your baby cannot have indomethacin (usually because of kidney or stomach problems) or if she has bleeding problems, the NICU doctors may recommend an operation to repair it. With your baby under a general anesthetic, a surgeon will close the PDA with a clip or a surgical stitch. This takes about an hour and babies usually do well afterward. Following her operation your baby will probably have a small tube draining any air leaks (see pneumothorax, page 61) away from her chest for a couple of days until the area begins to heal.

Outlook

Babies usually do well after their PDA closes or has been closed. However this heart condition can sometimes be a risk factor for long-term breathing problems.

Born at 24 weeks, in his first week of life John survived a pulmonary hemorrhage and a cardiac arrest, and then developed necrotizing enterocolitis. He is now a healthy three-year-old (see the photograph on pages 174-5).

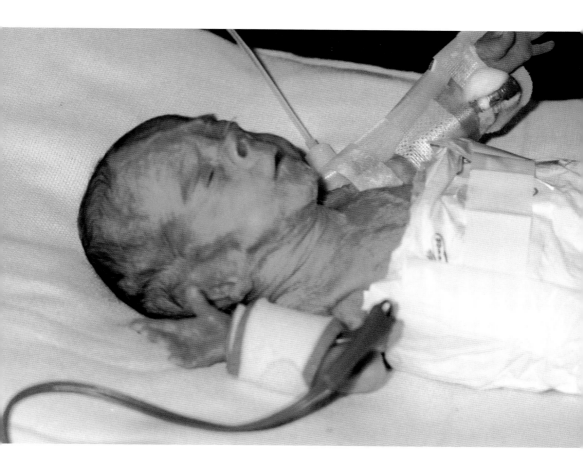

Breast milk helps to protect babies against developing NEC.

NECROTIZING ENTEROCOLITIS (NEC)

A potentially serious condition that affects the bowels of some newborn babies, necrotizing enterocolitis can occur when something is interfering with the blood flow to the baby's bowel, causing the area to die and then become infected.

NEC can be so mild that it can be cured simply by stopping feedings by mouth for your baby for a week or so and using IV feeding instead, to give the bowel a rest. However, at the other end of the scale, NEC can become severe enough to rupture the bowel wall and cause a serious infection called peritonitis in the abdominal cavity.

Premature babies are particularly vulnerable to NEC because they have immature digestive systems and a tendency to develop problems that prevent their blood from carrying oxygen throughout their body efficiently. There is no single cause of NEC, but anything that affects the smooth flow of your baby's blood can lead to asphyxia (too little oxygen getting to her tissues) and therefore to NEC. Risk factors include: sepsis; repeated apnea spells; not having grown very well in the uterus; the bowel not forming normally; low blood pressure; a cold virus; stress; patent ductus arteriosis; or moderate to severe bradycardia.

Symptoms

Babies with NEC can have a wide variety of symptoms, some of which can be quite subtle. This is why parents, who know their own baby better than anyone, may notice there is something not quite right even before the neonatal staff do. Important obvious signs are a bloated tummy and small amounts of blood in your baby's bowel movements. She may be vomiting, her food may stay in her stomach for longer than usual, or she might just be generally off-color, not wanting to feed and seeming tired and listless; and her temperature may be (even) less steady than usual. If your baby has severe NEC she will be very ill or listless, with a taut tummy and show signs of being in pain. Sometimes babies' limbs will also be swollen.

Since it can be difficult to tell for sure whether a baby has NEC, the doctors will probably order X-rays to check for any swellings in your baby's bowel or for the telltale gas bubbles. They would probably also check how much milk is getting left behind in your baby's stomach after feedings and test her bowel movements for traces of blood.

Treatment

The medical staff will stop your baby having any feedings by mouth. Instead, they will feed her either intravenously, or by using a tube that passes straight into her intestines below the site of the NEC, for up to a week or sometimes even longer. This will give the affected part of her bowel a rest from food and time to heal. They may also give antibiotics in case an infection has started and may put in a drain to take away any mucus that may have formed.

When feedings are introduced again, your baby should have breast milk, if possible, instead of formula. Breast milk is much easier to digest and contains enzymes and other special substances that can have healing effects on the intestinal lining itself. If giving breast milk is not possible, there is a special low-allergy milk formula that may be used instead.

Because a baby with NEC can become very ill quite rapidly she needs a close eye kept on her. This means she may have frequent X-rays, sometimes twice a day, to check that the bowel wall has not ruptured. She might also need some extra oxygen or ventilation in case of apnea or shock, and perhaps some extra fluids and medication to keep her blood pressure steady.

Surgery and its consequences

A baby with mild NEC will usually start to improve after a few days of antibiotics and IV feeding. However, if she does not start getting better fairly promptly or if there are signs that there is a bowel problem that might need to be repaired with surgery, her specialist may do an operation to look inside her abdomen to see what is happening.

Even if a baby has responded to treatment and recovered, she may still need surgery. Sometimes a baby's bowel can narrow around the NEC site as the area heals and produces scar tissue. Gut inflammation can also cause internal scarring. Either may create a blockage or

Short gut syndrome

Occasionally, so much of the bowel is affected by NEC and has to be removed that there is not enough left to absorb food, and it may be some time before the baby can take all her feeds by mouth once again. Until she can, she will be fed via an IV line (see page 26).

narrowing, though this can be put right quite easily with an operation.

Most seriously, if your baby's bowel has ruptured she will need emergency surgery to try to correct the problem by removing the damaged or scarred section of the bowel. Your baby may come back from the operating room with an ostomy—a narrow, open passageway from the bowel that ends in a small opening on the abdomen's surface called a stoma. The stoma has a small collection bag fitted carefully over it, which collects the baby's stools (feces). If the opening has been made into the large intestine it is called a colostomy; if it has been made into the small intestine, it is called an ileostomy. Both of these relieve the lower part of the bowel from its usual job of processing food and waste matter, and allow it more time to heal and grow.

Your baby's surgeon will carry out a second operation later on to join the ends of the now-healed-up bowel back together, and close up the stoma again.

Outlook

Good. Around three-quarters of babies with NEC get better just by being treated with antibiotics and having no feedings by mouth for a week. The problem sometimes recurs and the treatment has to be repeated. If a baby has surgery, this is usually successful. However, severe NEC is a very serious illness, and can sometimes be fatal.

If, after an operation to remove the damaged section, your baby's intestine is now too short to absorb enough nutrition from her food, she may need extra IV feeding, special milk formula and supplements for some months to make sure she is getting enough nutrients to grow healthy and strong. The bowel will usually regrow sufficiently to function properly but very occasionally an ostomy needs to be permanent.

Babies are usually only at risk of IVH in their first 2–3 days of life. However, an existing IVH "bruise" can get bigger for a few days after it forms. If a baby is three days old (or more) and has not had an IVH yet, he or she is very unlikely to have one.

INTRAVENTRICULAR HEMORRHAGE (IVH)

Any bleeding into the natural spaces in the brain, the ventricles, is called an intraventricular hemorrhage. Though this sounds worrying, it is very common in preterm babies, and it is usually so slight that, were it not for the routine brain scans carried out on very premature newborn babies, no one would ever know it had happened. The baby's system will tend to reabsorb any IVH blood naturally over the first few weeks, just as the blood from a bruise is absorbed back into your body.

IVH tends to happen because premature babies have a very rich blood supply to their brains, but this blood mostly flows through quite fragile capillaries. When the baby is being born, the strength of the blood flow and amount of oxygen reaching her brain changes many times, and may cause some of the weaker capillaries to break open and leak blood. Other possible causes can include anything that produces a major change in the brain's blood flow, such as severe BPD (see page 61).

Although IVH is generally harmless, occasionally it can be serious. Sometimes the bleeding may cause the

A nasogastric tube carries his food through his nose, down his throat to his stomach.

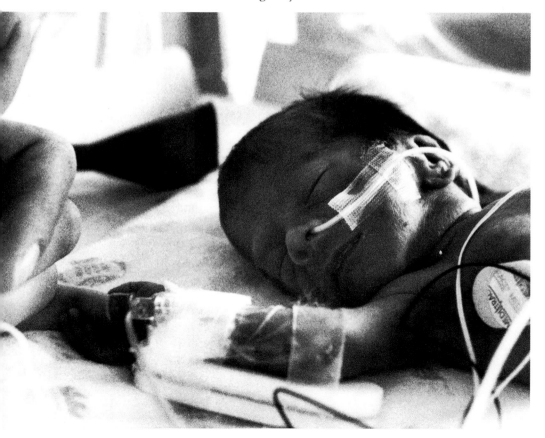

Hydrocephalus

Hydrocephalus is a condition in which the normal flow of cerebrospinal fluid around the brain is blocked (an IVH can cause such a blockage). The fluid builds up in the ventricles of the brain, which causes them to swell.

Hydrocephalus is sometimes referred to as "water on the brain."

Lumbar puncture

A procedure for removing some of the cerebrospinal fluid—the fluid that circulates around the spine and brain. This is kept inside a membrane which covers both brain and spinal column. A needle is passed gently into the lumbar region—the area at the base of the spine—piercing the membrane and drawing off some of the fluid.

brain ventricles to expand. Though that, too, often clears up leaving no trace that it has ever happened, it can have some longer-term side effects. For instance, there may be some bleeding within the tissue of the brain itself (this is called **hemorrhagic parenchymal infarction**. Again, a baby may show no sign of this at the time, but the brain cells die in the area where the hemorrhage occurred, leaving an empty space or cyst. Another possibility is that fluid may build up in the ventricles and cause them to swell.

Luckily, a cyst caused by IVH usually clears up of its own accord and any swelling dies away again. If so, the baby may well be none the worse for her IVH. However, in some cases premature babies may develop more serious difficulties such as cerebral palsy (see page 78), problems with hearing or sight, or learning difficulties. Severe IVH can be fatal.

Symptoms

If a baby does have more serious IVH, it can cause symptoms that may include apnea, bradycardia, anemia, seizures, floppiness and lethargy. The soft spot (called the fontanelle) on the top of her head may also bulge. A diagnosis of IVH will be confirmed by an ultrasound scan of the baby's head. This procedure can be done at her bedside if need be.

Treatment

Usually no treatment is needed for IVH. However, if fluid is building up in the ventricles, some of the extra fluid can be removed using a lumbar puncture, thus reducing the swelling. This may only be a temporizing measure. Occasionally, staff may give your baby medication that slows down the amount of fluid being made, again reducing the swelling.

Occasionally an IVH can cause build-up of fluid in the brain (hydrocephalus, see above) that does not clear either on its own or with medication. In these cases, the baby will have an operation to insert a small tube called a shunt, which removes the fluid as it is being made. This slim tube runs from the brain—going in just behind the ear—down under her skin to her abdomen, where the fluid is reabsorbed again.

A shunt is not nearly as cumbersome or noticeable as it sounds. When the baby develops more fat under her skin and grows more hair you cannot even see the tube. Sometimes the shunt may be temporary, but usually it will need to be permanent.

If the hemorrhage caused a good deal of blood to be diverted from her body's usual supply, your baby may be given a blood transfusion. If the IVH was a major one, the baby will probably have special physiotherapy and support to reduce its effects. Babies who have had anything other than a very mild IVH need to have a special hearing test while they are still on the NICU.

Outlook

If your baby has had an IVH that was marked enough to be noticed by her doctors, she will be followed up with regular check-ups so that any long-term problems that might possibly develop can be spotted early, and the most helpful treatments begun as soon as possible.

Developmental milestones Parents and doctors assess how a baby's development is coming along by seeing when the baby reaches specific developmental milestones, such as smiling, sitting without help, crawling, walking, saying her first words. If it does turn out that there is a problem, it may respond well to physiotherapy, speech therapy or special learning schemes.

Movement and muscle tone problems After an IVH a baby's movements can be jerkier and less well coordinated and her muscle tone can be too tense or too floppy. Movement or posture problems like this are often labeled as cerebral palsy (CP, see page 78) but they usually improve so much that they disappear on their own as the baby gets older. This is why a diagnosis of CP is tricky and cannot safely be made until a child is 12–18 months old, unless the CP is very severe. If muscle tone and control problems do not sort themselves out, they can usually be helped by physiotherapy.

Sight and hearing Some babies may develop sight or hearing problems (though most premature babies' hearing difficulties have nothing to do with IVH). If your baby has had an IVH she should have her hearing checked around the time she goes home. It is also possible that her vision may be slightly affected. The most common result is some form of a squint, which can usually be put right by eye specialists.

Seizures After a major IVH, a baby may occasionally have seizures—also commonly called fits or convulsions (see page 77)—for several months, even after she is well enough to go home. These can be treated successfully with drug therapy.

Hydrocephalus If your baby has a shunt to treat her hydrocephalus, this may sometimes become blocked, disconnected or cause an infection. Parents get to know the problem signs very quickly. An infection causes a temperature or reddening skin over the area where the shunt is, and if the tube is blocked or has disconnected, a baby may be abnormally sleepy, have jerkier movements, be especially irritable or have fits. If you are at all concerned, take your child to hospital to be checked; most potential problems can be stopped in their tracks by swift treatment.

RETINOPATHY OF PREMATURITY (ROP)

ROP is a disorder of the retina of the eye that usually only affects babies who are born at less than 32 weeks. Up to 30 percent of extremely premature babies (less than 28 weeks gestational age) will develop it to some degree. This is because though babies' eyes begin to form after only four weeks in the uterus, their retinas do not start developing until 28 weeks or so. Because eyes are the last sense organs to become complete, they are especially vulnerable to damage in babies who are born early.

How does ROP happen?

When the retina develops normally, it begins to grow a delicate, spiderweb network of tiny blood vessels, which starts at the center of the retina and spreads slowly outward. This process is finished a week or so after a baby is born, if she has gone to term. However, when a baby arrives prematurely, the retina's blood vessels do not have

The retina

The retina is a delicate ten-layer covering of special light-sensitive nerve cells coating the back of the eye. It registers the images that your eyes see and sends them flashing down the optic nerve, which runs from the retina to the brain, where they are "officially" recognized.

the chance to finish developing in the peace and dim light of the uterus, and have to do so in a harsher, usually brightly lit, environment instead.

If a baby develops ROP, this steady, symmetrical growth pattern—which looks like the fine, filigree roots of a young plant—is disrupted. The blood capillaries begin to grow too fast, and untidily. This can cause bleeding inside the eye and the formation of scar tissue, which pulls at the delicate retina. In severe cases, the retina comes away from the back of the eye altogether. This is rare, but it does sometimes happen; the condition is known as retinal detachment and means the baby will be partially blind.

There is no simple explanation for why these blood vessels develop oddly, but one of the main reasons seems to be too high levels of oxygen in the baby's bloodstream. Premature babies' systems are geared toward having exactly the right amount of oxygen to suit them at every stage of their development. In the uterus, this perfect amount is delivered directly into a baby's bloodstream by way of the placenta and umbilical cord. If a baby is born early, however, her breathing and regulatory systems may be too immature to ensure that absorbs the right amount of oxygen from whatever breathing method she is suddenly having to use—whether she is breathing in oxygen from the surrounding air naturally or receiving artificial help.

This may mean either that the baby can take in too much oxygen, or that she has trouble regulating the levels of it in her bloodstream. If she is getting too much oxygen, this may encourage the vulnerable, newly forming blood vessels in the retina to grow in a disorganized way. There are several risk factors for ROP that make sense if the excessive or fluctuating oxygen theory is true, including apnea, repeated blood transfusions, unstable blood pressure, IVH, patent ductus arteriosus, infections and multiple pregnancy (being one of twins, triplets or more).

Checking your baby's eyes

If your baby was born before she had spent 32 weeks in the uterus, she should have her eyes checked routinely by an eye specialist (ophthalmologist) every four to six weeks to

Some research suggests that bright light might cause eye damage in premature babies. Some NICUs are brightly lit by fluorescent tubing; in fact, in many NICUs the lighting has actually become five to ten times brighter over the past 20 years. Yet in the uterus, babies are in protective semi-darkness.

Many hospitals are now shading premature babies' eyes from glare, or keeping NICU lighting darker. Task lighting is used when nurses or doctors are examining or performing treatments on babies.

make sure the blood vessels in her retinas are developing normally. If there are any signs of ROP, the specialist will assess how mild or serious it is and how it is progressing, and will give whichever treatment is needed.

The eye examination is not thought to hurt, but it looks pretty uncomfortable. Some parents prefer to stay and soothe their baby while it is being carried out. Others feel they would rather not watch but make sure they are there immediately afterward to help settle their baby once again. The ophthalmologist uses eye drops to enlarge the baby's pupils so he can shine a light through them to see the retina behind. He also uses an instrument called a lid retractor to hold the eye open, plus another to push down gently on the white of the eye.

Treatment

Because ROP usually gets better of its own accord, your baby may not need any treatment, although doctors will keep a regular check on how her eyes are developing. If the ROP has progressed, it may need some minor surgery.

This may involve cryotherapy, which freezes the abnormal blood vessels to stop them growing. Cryotherapy is done with a tiny probe and liquid nitrogen as the freezing agent, under either a local or a general anesthetic. Your baby's eyes will be swollen for a few days afterward, but soothing ointments, eyedrops and cold compresses can all help.

The other method is laser treatment, which uses a tiny, powerful light beam to destroy the abnormal blood vessels. This treatment can be done under a light anesthetic, so there will be less of an anesthesia "hangover" afterward, and it also causes less discomfort and swelling. Lasers for ROP are still being tested out in several different hospitals worldwide.

Outlook

For around three-quarters of babies with mild ROP, there is no scarring or damage to the eyes. Some mild cases, however, do result in minor vision problems: these may mean that the child will need glasses—for near-sightedness, for example—or treatment with minor surgery and an eye-patch for crossed eyes (strabismus) or "lazy eye" (amblyopia).

SEIZURES

Also known as fits or convulsions, seizures happen when the brain's electrical systems short-circuit. A seizure is usually a sign that something is either irritating, or has damaged, the brain. Many babies who have seizures will only experience them mildly and briefly, but some have severe attacks again and again.

A seizure may occur because of an infection, imbalances in the usual substances found in the blood (for example, low blood sugar or calcium levels), after a major IVH or swelling of the brain (see hydrocephalus, page 72, and IVH, page 70) or as a consequence of an oxygen shortage or brain malformation. When no one can find out what is causing them, they are called idiopathic seizures.

Symptoms

The most obvious signs of a seizure are jerking movements of the body, stiffening of the arms, arching the back and flickering movements in the eyes, eyelids, mouth or tongue. There may be episodes of frantic sucking or apnea and/or bradycardia. Afterward the baby may be especially tired or sleepy for anything from a few minutes to a few hours.

Diagnosing a seizure can be tricky, however, because premature babies' movements are usually jerky until their nervous systems have matured. To check for seizures the doctors may have to carry out various tests. An electroencephalogram (EEG) will check out the electrical activity in your baby's brain. An ultrasound scan of the brain will show if there is any IVH swelling, or perhaps a malformation that could be causing the problems.

For a more accurate picture, a CT (computerized tomography) scan or an MRI (magnetic resonance imaging) scan may be carried out instead. Staff may also test your baby's blood or spinal fluid to see if there is an infection.

Normal jittery movements tend to stop if you place your hand gently on the baby's back, or cup her head and feet lightly; seizures, however, will not.

Treatment

If your baby is having seizures, she will be given anticonvulsant medication, such as phenobarbitone, which also acts as a calming sedative. However, this can cause lowered blood pressure and less easy breathing so staff should keep a careful watch on both.

Outlook

It is important to stress that most babies do recover completely from seizures and have no long-term ill effects. However, if the seizures happened because of severe oxygen shortage or a disease of the brain itself, they can continue to occur over a long period of time, and may be associated with a degree of brain damage. But whether this damage is caused by the oxygen shortage or brain disease, or by the convulsions, no one is quite sure.

If your baby has had repeated moderate-to-severe seizures, she will need regular follow-up visits to a neurologist or neonatologist to check her progress.

CEREBRAL PALSY (CP)

Cerebral palsy jumbles the messages that flash between the brain and muscles. If a child has CP, her brain is not controlling the muscles in the normal way. This may be because part of the brain is not working as it should, perhaps because it has been destroyed or has not developed properly.

Although in many cases there is no obvious reason for cerebral palsy, there are various possible causes. These include severe shortage of oxygen, perhaps as a result of a difficult or premature birth, IVH, or an infection during the first few weeks of pregnancy when the fetus was developing in the uterus (such as German measles). Very occasionally, CP may be caused by a rare genetic disorder. This can be inherited, even if neither parent has CP.

Symptoms

Initially, it is very hard to tell whether a premature baby has cerebral palsy, since between 40 and 80 percent of babies born early and weighing less than 3 pounds (1600g) do not have ordinary muscle tone or reflexes

There are three main types of cerebral palsy (CP):

1 **Spastic CP**, in which the child's muscles are stiff and it is harder for her to move her joints

2 **Athetoid CP**, in which the muscles change from being floppy to being tense in a way the child cannot control; she may also have speech and hearing problems

3 **Ataxic CP**, in which lack of control makes it difficult for the child to balance, and often causes jerky movement and speech

anyway at first. Jerky movements and poor muscle tone and posture are common in premature babies, but these problems have usually sorted themselves out by the time the child is 12 to 18 months old.

True CP only affects 3–6 percent of premature babies. Any problems a baby may have with movement or muscle control that look as if they might possibly be CP will need to be closely monitored for between 6 and 18 months before a pediatrician can be certain either way. The less severe the cerebral palsy is, the longer it takes to diagnose.

Usually it is the lower part of the baby's body that is affected. This can cause difficulties with balancing, sitting, walking and crawling, and also sometimes stiffness and muscle tightness in the legs. The intelligence of a baby with CP may be completely normal (and sometimes well

A sensor pad on the baby's foot monitors the level of oxygen in his blood.

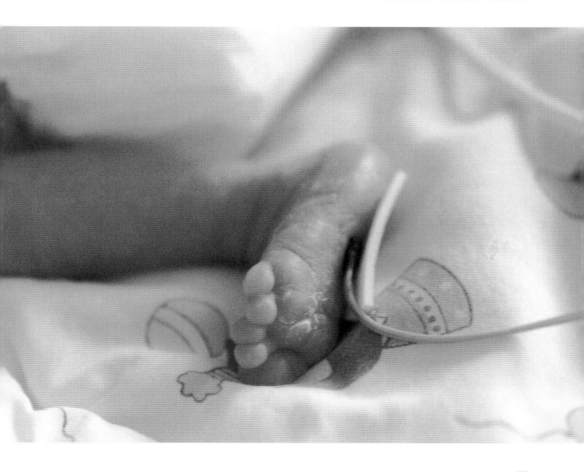

above average) but, as they grow older, some may have learning difficulties.

Treatment

Treatment includes physiotherapy to help your baby's muscle development and posture. If a baby's muscles are too stiff to work with, doctors may prescribe a drug called baclofen to relax the muscles. In some cases a baby with CP may also have an operation to correct any muscle tightness or contraction or any shortening of the muscles and ligaments that has developed, if these cannot be improved by exercise alone. For children who develop learning difficulties, there is a range of teaching methods that can be enormously helpful.

Outlook

The effects of CP can vary very widely, from the barely noticeable to the severely debilitating. If you want to know more about the likely effects as your baby grows, see pages 186–8. If you would like further specific information about CP, or just a listening ear, talk to your baby's nurse, pediatrician or neonatologist or seek out community support groups.

SERIOUS INFECTIONS

Some infections can arise as complications of a premature baby's illnesses or health problems. Two of the most serious are pneumonia and meningitis.

Pneumonia

Pneumonia is an acute infection of the lungs.

Symptoms Signs that your baby has a serious lung infection include difficulty in breathing or a change in the way she usually breathes, fluid in her lungs and an increasing number of apnea spells. To confirm pneumonia, the doctor will use a stethoscope to listen for the sound of fluid in your baby's lungs, and take an X-ray or perhaps extract a small sample of lung fluid via a tube so that the hospital lab can check for infection.

Treatment Your baby will be given a course of antibiotics (about five days long on average) either by IV or by injection. She may also have some extra oxygen, special nutrition and temperature control, and she might need support from a ventilator.

Outlook If pneumonia is spotted early and treated promptly, premature babies have an excellent chance of recovering completely. If not, it may lead to permanent lung damage or other serious infections, such as meningitis.

Meningitis

This is an infection or inflammation of the membranes covering the spinal cord or brain (the meninges). The infection may be viral or bacterial in origin.

Symptoms These can include many that are not unique to this illness, such as a baby having an increased number of apnea spells, a fluctuating heart and/or breathing rate, going off her food, arching her back and a tense fontanelle area. Doctors will confirm a diagnosis of meningitis by taking a small sample of her spinal fluid through a lumbar puncture (see page 72) for examination in the hospital lab.

Treatment Staff will give her antibiotics if the infection is bacterial and she may need extra intensive care, including ventilator support and extra oxygen, intubated nutrition (food by tube) and extra fluids and, if possible, around-the-clock, one-to-one nurse observation.

Outlook Usually the infection is spotted early and treated promptly, and babies make a good recovery. But if the treatment is not very successful meningitis can result in brain damage and nervous system complications. It also depends what type of meningitis it is as to how useful antibiotics are.

If a baby has had severe seizures or has been in a coma, there is a possibility of brain damage or even death.

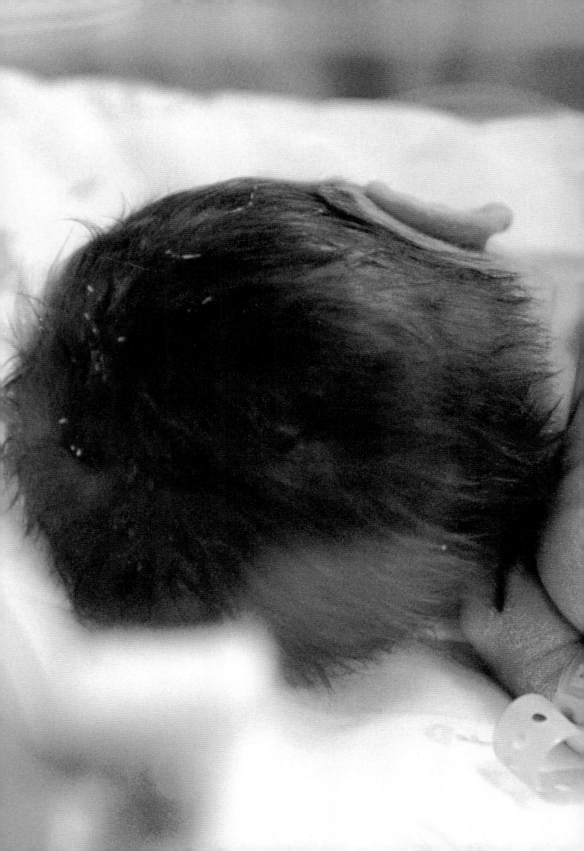

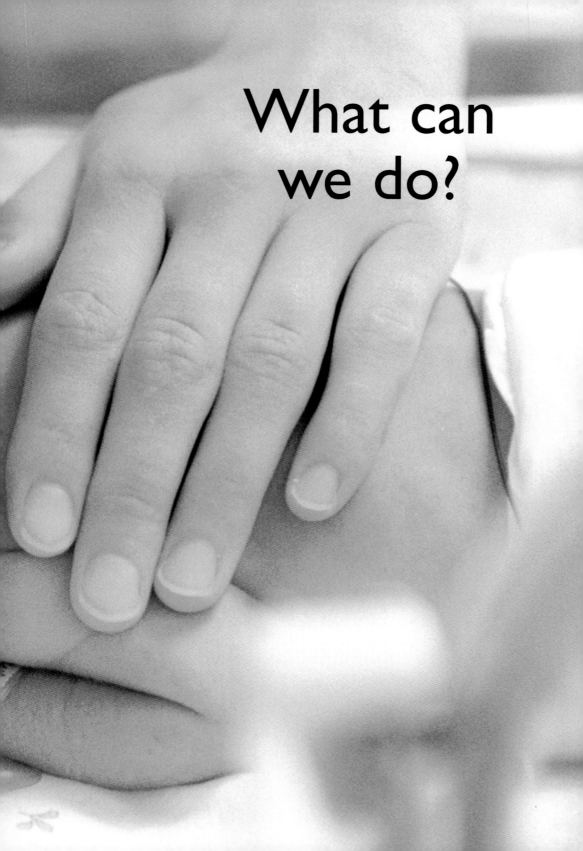

What can we do?

"I watched them for a while. They all looked like they knew just what they were doing. I felt so shaky and upset that I couldn't see what there might be for me to do too. So I just sat by Sacha."

Julie, mother of Sacha, born at 33 weeks

Many parents say that when they first came into the high-tech NICU and saw their babies surrounded by machinery and being cared for by busy, efficient neonatal nurses they felt intimidated, and almost as if they had been left out.

It may sometimes feel as though, because the nurses and doctors have taken charge of caring for your baby and seem to be doing it all so well, there is little you can really do to help. This could not be further from the truth. Just how hands-on you can be depends on how well your baby is, but there is an enormous amount both mothers and fathers can do every day, even for the most fragile of premature babies, and even while they are still in hospital.

STAFF AND PARENTS TOGETHER

Neonatal staff and parents can make a great team. This is because you can do vital things for your baby that the nurses cannot, and the nurses and doctors can help your baby in ways that you cannot.

Your baby already knows you

Parents' natural confidence can be shaken to its foundations by the shock of a premature birth and a baby who may be unwell, and need special care. Parents cannot believe that they already have their own special connections with their small son or daughter. And the barriers of special care, such as closed incubators, monitor leads and machinery, can make even the most confident mother or father feel cut off from their child. But if you are his mother, your baby has until very recently been physically sharing your body. Research shows that while a baby is in his mother's uterus, mother and baby are so closely connected that the baby can even be aware of his mother's moods.

Mothers are the people that new babies know best in the world. It may sound odd to say your baby already knows you, especially if at the moment he is very premature or unwell and it seems as if he is not responding much to anything, even when you sit beside him or talk to him. Yet your baby already knows your voice. He will have been born knowing it because he has spent many hours hearing you talk, laugh, sing and shout while you carried him in your uterus. The sound may have been muffled but it was *yours* and so it is *your* voice that has more power to comfort and reassure him than anyone else's.

Why your baby needs you

Mothers and fathers can give their baby their undivided attention, protection and care. You are the only people who are there entirely for your baby or babies: nurses' care has to be shared. You are the one constant factor in your baby's life.

And mothers can make breast milk. This is so good for premature babies that it amounts to a valuable part of their medical treatment (see page 69).

Working together to support your baby.

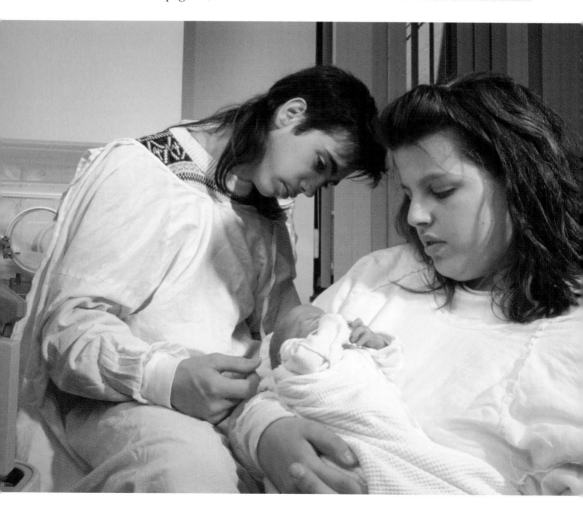

Nurses change at every shift: parents don't.

More importantly, you are the only people who can give your baby love: you can comfort and soothe him and give him your time. In fact, parents are their baby's best comforters—just being there for him can have a positive effect on his health. Neonatal staff say that they have often seen the level of oxygen in premature babies' systems rise when their mothers or fathers came to sit beside them, even though the babies had not opened their eyes nor the parents said a word.

You are also the ones who know your baby best. It may not seem so at first, but when you have spent more time with your baby you will find that, despite all the medical expertise surrounding him, you know him. This is partly because you have the time to spend sitting by him and watching him day after day: nurses do not have the time to do this. Because of this, you are usually the first to know if your baby is unwell or if he is getting better, and whether he is comfortable, coping with what is happening to him or is getting distressed. You are also your baby's best advocates and protectors. All this makes a great difference to how well he is cared for.

"Trust yourself. You know more than you think you do."

Dr Benjamin Spock

BABYWATCHING: UNDERSTANDING YOUR BABY'S SIGNALS

One of the most important—and most natural—things you can do is to understand your baby. Many parents say they feel helpless, especially if their baby is very unwell, and all they can do is just sit by his incubator, but this is the perfect place to be to get to know your baby—the better to understand his own personal signals and body language.

You may think that because your baby is not yet mature enough to cry or smile you will not be able to understand what he is feeling. Yet even though he has been born too early and his body is very small, he is sending you many different, definite messages. He can do this without crying, without words, sometimes without even moving.

All babies, including premature babies, use body language and facial expressions to tell you how they are or what they need. This is not an exact language, but it offers

When your baby

★ has a bright, shiny alert look in his eyes

★ is making "ooh" shapes with his mouth

★ can pay attention—perhaps only for a few seconds—to something such as your face, a moving toy, your voice

★ is trying to lift his head or turn, as you hold him against your shoulder

he is happy and may be ready for some interaction with you

valuable clues to what your baby is feeling. And as almost any neonatal nurse will tell you, it's usually you—your baby's mother or father—who can read your own baby the best, partly because you are his parent, and partly because you spend far more time sitting beside him and watching over him than anyone else.

There is no such thing as a definitive guide to the way premature babies communicate. Each baby is a unique individual and the meaning of the signals your baby gives you depends a good deal on how many weeks he spent in the uterus before he was born and how mature, and how well, he is at the moment. It can also depend on how he is being cared for, what medication he is receiving (some types can have a sedating effect) or whether he is on a ventilator.

"You cannot say a newborn baby does not talk. It is we who do not listen."

Frederick Leboyer, obstetrician and natural childbirth pioneer

When your baby brings his hand up to his face it is a good sign. He is able to comfort himself without waiting for you to do it for him.

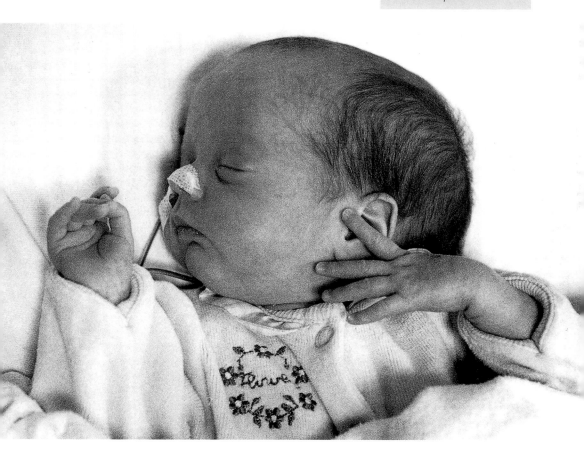

When your baby

★ is lying with his arms and legs relaxed

★ looks alert, his eyes open and shiny

★ has a smooth, relaxed face —not taut, no lines or furrows

★ has tried to curl himself over sideways

★ has pink, even skin color

(And, in a more mature premature baby—)

★ is looking at you, or at something, with interest (rather than staring fixedly)

★ may be trying to smile

he's showing that he's feeling comfortable.

When your baby tries or manages to

★ clasp his hands together

★ bring his hands up to or near his mouth or face

★ suck on his fingers or hands

★ hold onto the corner of his blanket

★ have his feet touching, one on top of the other

★ tuck himself into a cozy, curled-over position

★ turn his gaze or head away

he's showing he can comfort himself.

Some signals can have different meanings at different times. As you watch them, try to think what—knowing, as only you do, your baby's particular and special circumstances—they might mean. If your baby yawns or hiccups, for instance, this may be a way of breaking away from something that is happening to him because he can no longer cope with it, or it may mean that he is becoming slightly short of oxygen. Or, of course, a yawn may simply mean that he is tired.

Interpreting the clues

All the signs need a bit of interpreting. It may take a parent or an expert neonatal nurse to know whether a baby is lying in a relaxed way or is just plain tired out. And it may take time to realize that if your baby turns his gaze or his head away when you are looking at his face, talking gently to him or stroking him, this is a positive sign. It is not a rejection of you; it may merely mean that he needs a rest just at this moment, and is mature enough now to be able to break contact in this way—or he may have noticed something interesting over there. A very sick or very immature baby might not be able do this.

Premature babies often drop—alarmingly abruptly—into a sudden light sleep, but that usually just means they have had enough and so they have shut the world out. If your baby does this you might feel he would like to be put back in his crib for a rest, or he might prefer you to hold him quietly, shading his eyes, until he wakes again.

Positive signs

There are many positive signs. For example, when you see your baby showing any of the signs listed above left, it probably means that he is feeling comfortable. If he is doing—or even trying to do—any of the things listed below left it means that he can, or is trying to, comfort himself, without having to wait for you or a nurse to see what is needed and do it for him.

Making it easier

However, if you notice your baby trying to do any of these things listed but not quite making it, you can help him succeed. Perhaps he is taking what look like swipes at his face, but you feel he is really trying to get his fingers into his mouth—you can help by gently bringing his fingers up to his mouth. Are your baby's fingers moving over or scrabbling at his blanket? He may be trying to hold it for comfort—slide a corner into his hand for him to hold.

Signs that your baby might like help

If your baby has scooted down into the corner of his incubator he may have done this because he didn't like all that space around him—it may feel very empty after being in the uterus. Perhaps he could have some soft nesting (see pages 93–4) around him as boundaries to make him feel secure? He may also need this if he stretches out his legs to touch the sides, but sometimes it may be that he just likes to stretch.

A yawn can be a sign that he needs more oxygen—or he may just be tired.

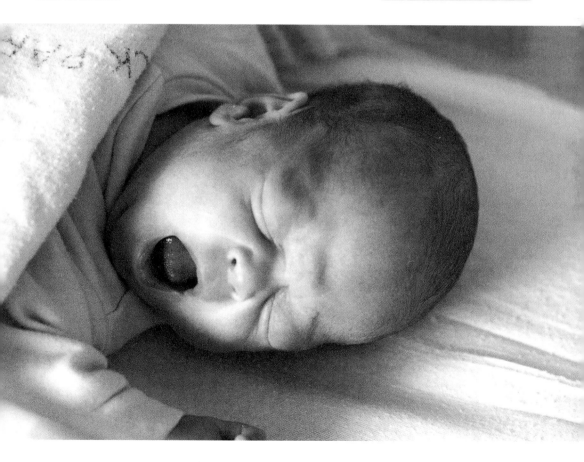

When your baby

★ has stiff or tense arms, legs or body

★ has a stressed or taut look on his face

★ is being frantically active and cannot seem to calm down

★ has a mottled, paler, dusky or very red skin color

★ is breathing fast and/or his heartbeat has suddenly speeded up

something is either physically not right or is bothering him.

Changes in heartbeat and breathing

It is normal for the heartbeat and breathing rate of premature babies to speed up and slow down, sometimes several times a day. This will stop when their circulatory and nervous systems settle down and mature, unless they have a long-term problem that needs treatment. Your baby's doctors and nurses would soon notice if he did have a problem, and would make sure he had the medical or surgical treatment he needed.

Frowning may just mean he is concentrating, but grimacing or making a face usually means he is not happy about something and would like some help. If his eyes are dull, this may be because his systems are very immature, it may mean that he is in pain—or it may just be that he wants to go to sleep.

Usually if your baby has a panicky expression in his eyes, with his gaze "locked" on something, this means that he is having difficulty in coping with whatever is happening to him at the moment, but cannot seem to pull away from it on his own. In this case he may need you to help him by cutting back on anything disturbing or stimulating him by perhaps tucking him up cozily in his incubator and shading his eyes, or (as far as possible) quieting any noise going on nearby, or just holding him quietly, without rocking or moving. Some babies, however, also use this "locked" gaze as a way of calming themselves.

Signs of trouble

In the column on the left are some signs that may suggest that something is physically not right—though, again, it may simply be that your baby is having difficulty coping with whatever is happening to him at the moment. If you see any of these signs, ask a nurse if they could come and check him with you.

OBSERVING AND INTERPRETING YOUR BABY

Even the youngest premature babies are born with their own distinctive personalities, their own likes and dislikes. One may like his feet being lightly held, another may get upset if she is not partially covered up when his diaper is changed, one may be placid, another irritable.

As his parents, you are probably the people who spend most time with your baby. Have you seen how he reacts to having his diaper changed, a blood test taken, his breathing tube suctioned if he is on a ventilator? What helps calm him down when he is upset? What seems to make him comfortable? Have you noticed that anything in particular seems to upset him?

Detailed observation like this can give everyone vital information about the best way to handle your baby, so tell his nurses what you have noticed.

PROTECTING YOUR BABY'S SLEEP

Plenty of sleep is very important in helping a premature baby grow, especially if they have not been well. Unfortunately they often don't get it because they tend to be disturbed too often. These disturbances include staff carrying out medical procedures, noise, lights that are too bright, alarms going off on equipment, the unit's telephone, even the buzzer on the NICU door.

There are several things you might like to try to protect your baby from disturbance. You can ask if people

Some parents have found it useful to hang a notice on their baby's incubator to help the medical staff understand him. On it they put details about the baby, such as his name and who his parents are; what he likes (for example, being shaded from bright lights); and what he doesn't like (such as loud voices talking across his incubator).

A sheet draped over the top of the incubator shields the baby's eyes from the bright lights of the NICU.

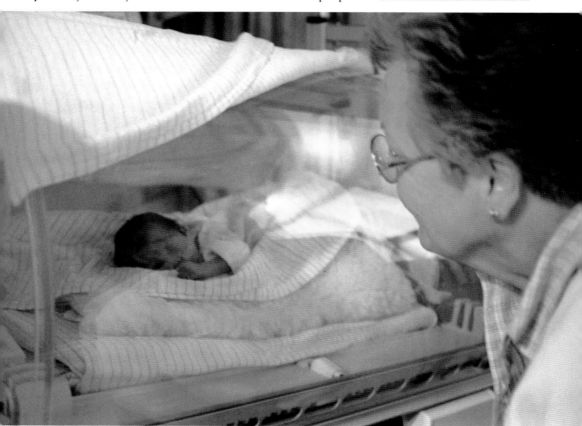

Tips for keeping your baby undisturbed

★ Turn off any lights near your baby when they are not being used.

★ Ask for a screen to shield your baby if he is near another baby who is receiving phototherapy.

★ Pad any drawer under the incubator, or nearby cupboard, that keeps banging.

★ If your baby's incubator is in earshot of the unit's shrilling telephone or door buzzer, ask to move him somewhere quieter or to turn down the phone's ring to a softer level, or ask whether the phone could be replaced with one that does not ring out loud but instead has an alarm that lights up.

Movement and posture problems affecting their ability to support their own heads and to sit up unaided are very common in premature babies. In their first year at least 40 percent—and possibly up to 80 percent—of premature babies born weighing less than 3½lb (1600g) are affected. Good positioning can help prevent these problems from developing.

could talk very softly when they are near your baby and he is sleeping and put a sign on his crib asking for quiet, to remind them. Find out from the medical staff whether regular interventions, like blood sampling or diaper changing, could be scheduled together as much as is practical, so your baby has chunks of peace and quiet, and also whether it is possible for him to have a nap in the morning and one in the afternoon when doctors and other caregivers do not disturb him for check-ups and tests unless they are urgent. Some units have a system of quiet periods, often in the afternoon. During these quiet times, only parents can handle and be with their babies, unless there is an emergency. Premature babies ideally need quiet hours during the day and night.

PROTECTING YOUR BABY'S EYES

A baby's eyes are the last sensory organs to develop. This means that they are the most immature organs at birth, even for term babies. It makes sense, therefore, to protect premature babies' eyes until they have had a chance to mature. NICUs are usually brightly lit places, however, though some are moving to keeping them dimmed at all times. Research suggests that, in some cases, the lighting levels are up to a third higher than recommended, and some studies further indicate that this may be associated with damage to premature babies' vulnerable, still-developing eyesight. On the other hand, staff take a risk that, if they cover the incubator to protect against bright light, they could fail to spot problems with the baby or the equipment inside, such as a blockage in a vital tube.

Some NICUs use padded incubator covers, because it is thought they help protect premature babies' immature eyes from possible damage from bright lighting, and also help them rest. The padding reduces noise levels too.

Partial covering

Some NICUs take the middle route, partially covering some of the incubators so the babies' heads are in shade but their bodies and any monitor wires or tubing are still under bright light and so easy to check. This method of partial shading is recommended by some specialists, especially if the baby is medically unstable or critically ill. So if your baby's unit does not cover the incubator you could suggest that a blanket or baby quilt be draped over at least the top half of the crib.

POSITIONING: HOW TO HELP YOUR BABY LIE COMFORTABLY IN THE INCUBATOR

If you look at the way a premature baby lies in his incubator, then at the way a newborn term baby lies, you may notice that term babies often lie in a curled-up position, tucked around themselves. But premature babies have weak muscle tone and, if they are not supported in any way and left on their backs, they tend to sprawl, legs akimbo and arms flung out sideways. Many parents feel

Disturbed rest

Research has shown that, in most neonatal units, babies are disturbed every 4 to 10 minutes.

Rolled-up flannelette offers support to the baby while helping him feel secure.

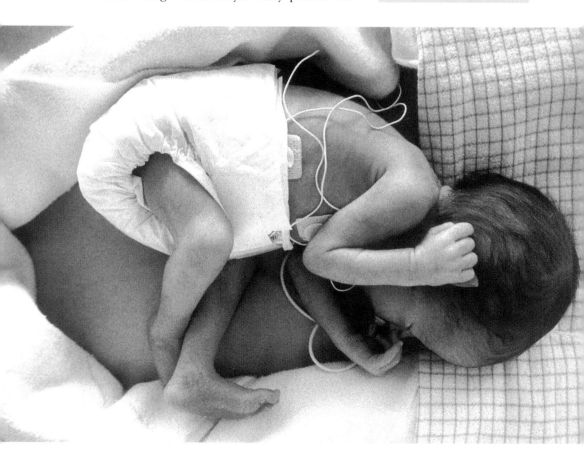

Positioning tips

* Place soft supports for his hips, knees, shoulders, neck and side.
* Change his head position regularly.
* Raise the head end of his incubator to a 30-degree angle.
* Change the position he lies in from time to time.
* Nest him.
* Place soft boundaries around him to encourage him to flex against them.
* Bring his hands up close to his mouth.
* Put him in the balanced "midline" position, again bringing his hands up near his mouth.
* Read his body language to check he is comfortable.
* Place him lying on his front; this may help if your baby is finding it difficult to breathe.

instinctively that it is uncomfortable for their babies to lie like this. There is no specific scientific evidence for that, but it certainly looks uncomfortable.

There is a growing amount of medical research, however, that suggests that if premature babies are helped and supported to lie in better positions, this can help them develop normal posture and muscle tone. This is important because it means that they will be far more likely to sit, crawl, walk and move their arms and legs normally as they grow up—these are things that premature babies do tend to have problems with (see page 186–7). Both nurses and parents can help with positioning. This is the practical art of gently supporting premature babies so that they lie in the best and most comfortable positions in their incubators. Positioning helps babies to lie in ways that are likely to be comfortable, but also encourages them to practice gently flexing their muscles, or to push against boundaries. This in turn helps their bodies to develop normally.

Flexion

Babies who have been born too early have not yet had the opportunity to build up enough strength or muscle tone to lie comfortably in a flexed position (curled over) or to support themselves, as a term baby does. The usual way that babies develop some muscle tone is by pushing their arms, legs, hands, feet and shoulders against the walls of the uterus from time to time—a kind of "working out" in the uterus. Neonatal staff call this flexion. The bigger a baby grows, the less space he has in the uterus, the more he flexes against its walls and the more muscle tone he develops. This is partly why the earlier a baby is born, the less muscle strength and tone he has.

How to position a baby

You can use soft rolls of flannelette baby sheets, small foam shapes or even mini bean bags to support your baby's small body. These aids also give a baby something to flex against. There are also specially made supports from specialist manufacturers, but these are more expensive. The supports may be placed at all or any of the following places: hips, back, shoulders, knees, or neck.

NICU staff may also nest a baby by tucking a roll of fabric all the way around the body. This means that he can be supported to lie in the best position for encouraging good posture and muscular development, and to feel comfortably contained and secure, as he used to be in the uterus. A nest will also give him something to push his feet against, or support his arms so he can bring his hands up to his mouth more easily.

Premature babies are not usually keen on having a lot of space around them and some have repeatedly been found in the corner of their incubators if they are strong enough to inch their way down there. If your baby likes to do this, let him be. He will waste more energy trying to

Overheating

If a baby is very premature and finds it especially hard to control his own body temperature, he needs to be checked very regularly to make sure that the nesting materials are not making him too hot.

Gently turning a baby's head at regular intervals can help prevent head flattening.

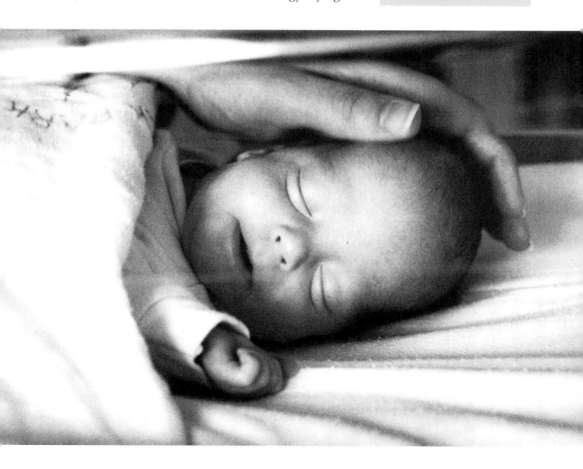

Front or back at home?

It is completely safe for a baby to sleep on his front in the NICU, where he is closely monitored all the time. However, when you take your baby home, it is much safer for him to sleep on his back (see pages 171–172). This is why many NICUs will begin getting babies who have been happily sleeping on their fronts in hospital used to sleeping on their backs before they go home.

Sometimes a gentle touch is the most a parent can do.

find the boundaries he is searching for if he is constantly being repositioned.

How good positioning can help your baby

Not only can this help develop normal movement and posture, it can also make a baby's breathing easier and encourage a regular heartbeat. Being supported in a more comfortable position can help promote regular sleeping patterns.

It is also an aid to good digestion: placing a premature baby so he is supported comfortably on his right side can help reduce gastric reflux (GER), a common problem for premature babies (see page 166).

Good positioning helps prevent the unhappy, and sometimes frantic, fidgeting that neonatal staff call "purposeless movement". Premature babies can become

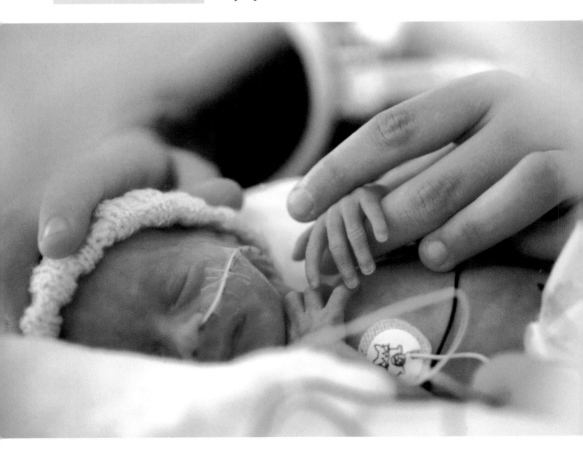

surprisingly agitated, moving around a good deal when they are distressed or uncomfortable, and this uses up energy and calories that the babies need for growing and recovery. The more comfortable and well supported a baby is, the less he will fidget, the less stressed he is likely to be, and the faster he will gain the weight he needs.

Preventing head flattening

Careful positioning can also avoid "head flattening." The development of a slightly misshapen head and face is quite common in babies and toddlers who have been born very early, before 28 weeks. It can happen because the bones of a premature baby's skull are still quite soft, so that when his relatively large head presses down (quite heavily, because he has weak neck muscles) against the surface he lies on, this can press his skull slightly out of shape. The result can be a flattening of the back or sides of the head, and a high narrow forehead and eyes that seem to be placed more to the sides than is usual.

To prevent head flattening, the baby's head needs to be turned regularly, although there is no agreement yet on exactly how often. Some units do this every two hours, some every six. Some also alternate placing a baby on his back to sleep with placing him on his front. Various aids are also used, though, again, there are no firm conclusions yet about which work best. They include water pillows, water beds, soft air-filled mattresses and soft donut-shaped head supports. If you are concerned about head-flattening, ask your baby's medical staff what they recommend to help prevent this.

Front or back?

It also matters whether your baby is laid on his front (prone), back (supine), side or a mixture of all three. Most neonatal units used to nurse sick premature babies on their backs. This was partly so that the staff could see quickly and easily how they were, and partly because it was easier to position NICU equipment such as umbilical catheters and ventilator tubes. However, over the last few years many research studies have suggested that premature

Therapeutic Touch by parents

1 Sit down by your baby, preferably at a time when he is fairly settled, not due to be handled, for example for diaper changing or any medical tests, and not hungry, and the NICU is fairly quiet. Look at him and focus all your attention on him. Try—as one nurse trained in Therapeutic Touch put it—to "send him your love, with your eyes." Do this for a few moments—as long as feels right to you.

2 Now hold one of your hands, palms down, about 2–4in (5–10cm) above your baby's head, and the other a similar distance from his feet. You could use your fingers for this instead if you feel that your palms are "too big" for your tiny baby. Try to send him your love through your hands or fingers.

3 If you would like to do a little more, try slowly "stroking" your baby from his head to his feet, again keeping your hands 2–4in (5–10cm) away from his body. Do this for as much time as you feel is right. There is no set "correct" length of time.

4 To finish, bring your hands or fingers back to their original position, just above your baby's head and feet, let them stay there for a few seconds, then end.

Holding him close

babies used up too much energy, and had lower levels of oxygen in their blood, when they were laid on their backs.

There are major advantages to babies' sleeping on their fronts. These include using up less energy (premature babies have little to spare), spending more time asleep, less fidgeting and restless movement (which again helps save what little energy they have for recovery and growing), a slower heart rate and more stable breathing. There is also evidence that raising the head end of a baby's mattress to a 30-degree angle helps his digestion, lungs and heart to work better.

THERAPEUTIC TOUCH

Despite its name, this is a no-touch method of "massage" that uses the natural healing energy from a parent's or nurse's hands held roughly 2–4 inches (5–10cm) or so away from the baby's body. It is something parents can try on even the very smallest premature baby, and therapeutic touch can often be used for babies who are too fragile or unwell to be massaged, even very lightly, in the usual way.

Therapeutic touch (sometimes called healing touch) may sound a bit strange and "New Age," but it is well accepted by many nurses and has become more accepted at some medical centers in the U.S. and Canada. Its benefits are backed up by clinical research trials, though only one or two have been carried out specifically on premature babies in NICUs. In North America more than 80 universities use and teach the therapy. According to clinical trials, the technique appears to have a deep relaxing effect, can reduce pain, soothe anxiety and distress, and may also help wounds and injuries heal faster.

You could ask a nurse trained in this type of no-touch massage to do it for your baby. But you can also easily learn how to do it yourself. As the mother or father of your baby, you are an especially good person to do this because you love your child so much, and know him better than anyone else.

Some parents find they prefer a bit of temporary privacy when they use therapeutic touch for their baby, and ask if they might have some screens around them for a little while.

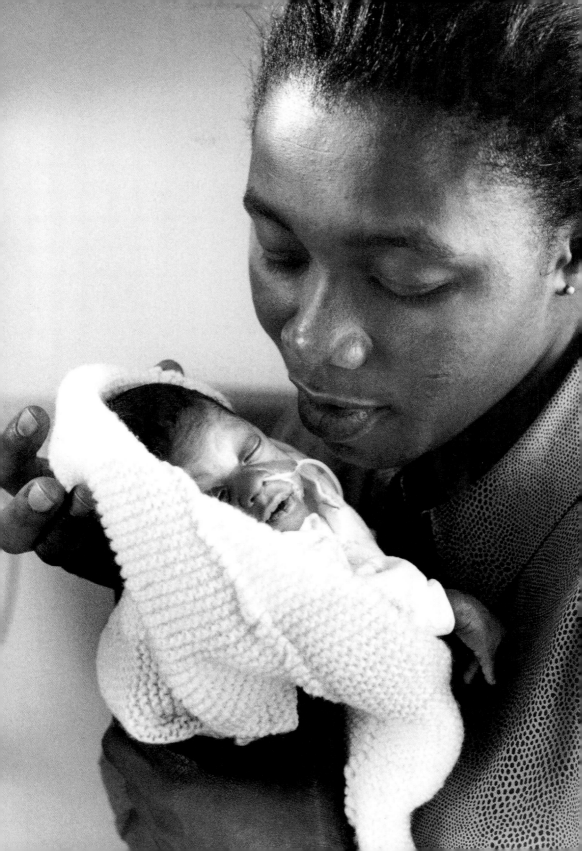

10 baby-comforting ideas

★ Reduce any stress from his surroundings (for example, from noise or bright light).

★ Make sure he is lying supported in a comfortable position in his cot.

★ Put your hands gently on his bottom or back if he is frantic or restless.

★ Cup one hand gently around his head, the other gently touching his feet.

★ Swaddle him (with his arms free) and lay him on his side in his incubator with some kind of cover shading his eyes.

★ Hold him close without rocking or talking.

★ Speak softly to him without making eye contact.

★ "Think" calm, love and energy into him.

★ Give him your little finger to suck or hold.

★ Wrap him in a blanket and hold him quietly.

★ Place him comfortably within a cozy "nest" of soft rolls of bedding (check that he doesn't get too hot).

CONTAINMENT CARE

This is another kind of treatment you might like to try, if your baby is not ready for even the gentlest massage just yet. With containment care you cup your hand around your baby's head, without quite touching it. Leave your hand in position, and imagine warmth and energy flowing from your hand into his head.

You can take this further when you feel your baby is ready (check with your baby's nurses or doctors): cup your hand around his head just touching it, gently cradling his feet with your other hand.

Even the tiniest premature babies usually like this. This may be because it gives them a sense of being safely held in a limited space, as they were in the uterus.

COMFORT AND CONTACT

Almost all parents of even the tiniest or most fragile of premature babies have a powerful instinct to stroke, lay their hands upon, and soothe their own infants. Mothers or fathers will get to know instinctively just the sort of contact their baby needs, or can cope with. There are many things a parent can do to make contact with their premature baby, even when he is too fragile or unwell to be picked up and cuddled.

Talking to your baby

Talking to your baby gently and quietly is a very natural thing for any parent to do, and is an excellent and effective way of making contact with your baby, no matter how young he is. If he shows any signs—such as yawning or turning his head—that he is finding this attention too much to cope with, leave it for a bit and try again later, using your baby's responses as your guide (see page 86).

Placing your index finger gently in his hand

Even extremely premature babies can grasp with their hands (although strong grasp reflexes do not come until a baby is 32 weeks or more, and actual muscle tone tends to develop relatively late, from 34–36 weeks) and they find it comforting to have something to hold on to. In the uterus, from about 24 weeks on, their hands are big enough to grasp the umbilical cord; ultrasound pictures of babies this age often show them doing so. Some researchers have suggested that this is a baby's first comforter, and that even when he is still in the peace of the uterus, it helps him feel more secure. Holding your finger may bring that feeling back, as well as giving him precious physical contact with you.

Letting him suck the tip of your little finger

Babies of all ages find sucking very soothing. Your baby will have been practicing sucking movements since he was only 11–12 weeks old in your uterus, and a few weeks after that he may have coordinated his thumb into his mouth, as many ultrasound scan pictures show. If you find that your baby likes to suck on your little finger, make sure the nail is very short with no sharp edges anywhere, and that nails and hands are very clean.

However, being able to suck on your finger does not necessarily mean he is ready to breast- or bottle-feed yet. To do this he needs to be able to coordinate his sucking, breathing and swallowing.

Gently bringing his hands near his mouth

This encourages him to suck his own fingers and thumbs. Finger and thumb sucking is a really important part of his learning to comfort and calm himself, rather than having to wait for you or a nurse to do the comforting for him. Now that he is outside the uterus, your baby might not yet be able to coordinate his movements accurately enough to bring his fingers to his mouth, but it is a good thing if he is trying.

Comforting your baby during interventions

"Interventions" is a catch-all term for anything that involves touching your baby. This could range from a cuddle or a massage to having an IV line or a feeding tube inserted.

As NICUs have become more high-tech, the number of times premature babies are handled in an average day has increased dramatically. The hospital staff have to do these things to care for your baby and to check on his well-being. Unfortunately, many necessary interventions are

"At first I used to feel stupid, leaning over a 33-week-old premature baby and saying something like 'Look sweetheart, Mum's really sorry but you have to have this blood test done now. I know it isn't very nice but it will only be for a moment … there, it's OK now…' just as you would for an older baby or toddler. But then I thought: who's to say an older baby understands you word for word, but that doesn't stop most parents chatting away to them, does it?"

Valerie, Lee's mother

"I was grateful to all the nurses, I really was. They were being so kind to us, and they had saved Gail's life. But when I saw them doing all these things for her, even kissing her head and stroking her back to soothe her—I felt sick with jealousy, and anger. That was my baby. How dare those other women stroke the top of her head like that? Then tell me she was still too fragile to be picked up by me, her mother?"

Jo, mother of Gail, born at 31 weeks

thoroughly uncomfortable. Some hurt. And all of them may be disturbing for your baby.

You can lessen the impact of the unpleasant interventions by comforting your baby as they happen, helping to settle him afterward. Parents usually have far more time to do this than nurses do, and because you know your own baby best you will be able to soothe him better than anyone.

Some parents like to be there to support their baby through interventions and to help him settle afterward. Others find that they themselves can become upset when they see their baby distressed. If this is the case for you, would you perhaps be able to help your baby most by not being there during the procedure itself, but coming to comfort and soothe him immediately afterward instead? You may find that whether or not you stay with your baby throughout depends on how you yourself are feeling, how tired you are, how well or unwell your baby is, and on what sort of intervention is being carried out. Follow your feelings and your own instincts. Just do whatever feels right to you at each particular time.

You can comfort your baby by talking to him for a minute or two before the intervention happens. Some parents find they like to talk to their baby as if he were a much older child. They explain quietly what will happen, and that it won't last long. Your baby may well catch your drift and appreciate it, even though he will not understand your actual words.

During the intervention you could give your baby your finger to hold or suckle on, cup a hand around his head, put a reassuring hand against his back, or gently touch his arm or hand. Afterward it is important to soothe him until he is calm and relaxed again. Premature babies have not yet developed the skills they need to calm themselves back down after being upset. They are what NICU staff call "disorganized", meaning that their nervous systems are not yet developed enough for them to return quickly to normal after something has upset or disturbed them. They need your help to do this.

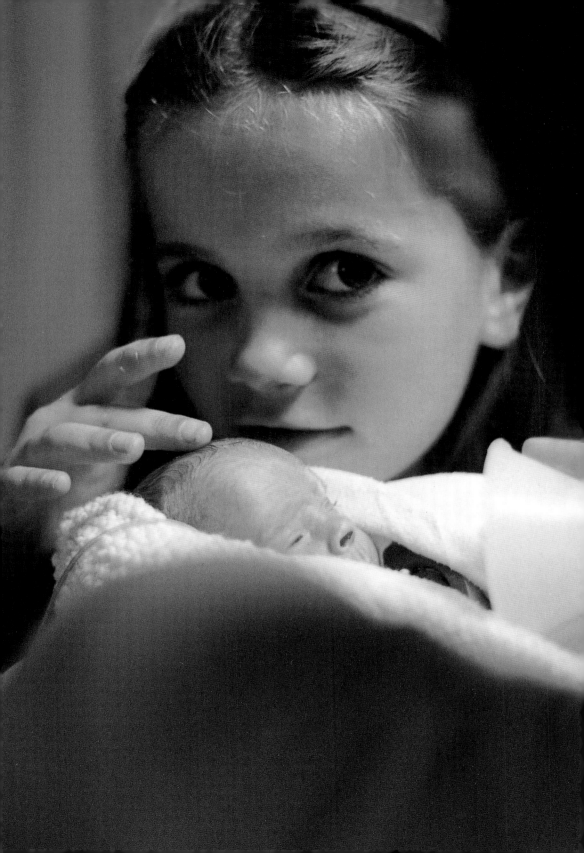

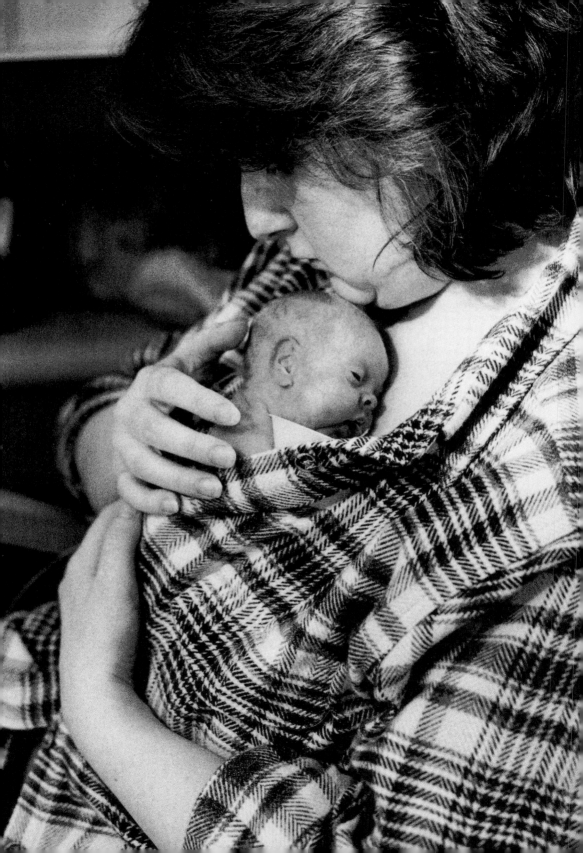

HOLDING YOUR BABY

You can hold even the tiniest of premature babies from 24 or 25 weeks, so long as they are medically stable—that is: though they may be ill, they are holding steady and not getting any worse. If you want to hold your own baby for a little while, it is your right to do so. Do not take no for an answer if staff seem reluctant, unless there is a good medical reason why your child must not be disturbed at all for the moment. Talk to your baby's pediatrician or neonatologist about this if you are not sure whether your baby is medically stable or not, or if you are still not being encouraged to hold him.

When they're all wired up. . .

Many parents have said that though they wanted very much to hold their babies properly, they found it quite alarming the first couple of times.

Don't worry if a tube comes out while you are holding or picking up your baby—that's always happening. Some neonatal nurses say that it often seems as if one of premature babies' favorite occupations is pulling their tubes out by themselves. There is no need to panic as it is really not much of a problem, nor is it a bar to lifting your baby out yourself. Just call a nurse and she will put the tube back in again.

KANGAROO CARE

Kangaroo care is a way of holding your premature baby so that she rests on your chest, with her bare skin against yours. It can be very good—from a medical point of view—for the babies themselves. It can be good for parents too because it feels close and loving: it means you can have some real physical contact with your baby and it offers a gentle, hands-on way of really mothering or fathering your own child.

Babies can be held this way even when they are very small and premature. The most important factors affecting whether your baby can have kangaroo care are whether: your baby is medically stable (see page 106); the NICU nurses are familiar with this way of holding a premature

How to give kangaroo care

Wear something that unbuttons down the front, and wash your hands, to cut down the possibility of infection.

1 It is a good idea to put a cotton bonnet on your baby if he is not already wearing one —babies lose a lot of heat from their heads; but take off the rest of his clothes, or at least undo them at the front.

2 Undo the front of your clothes, lift your baby from his incubator and lay him on his tummy between your breasts (fathers should lay their baby on their chests).

3 Your baby's position is very important: so that he can breathe easily, he needs to lie on his tummy and upright against you, with his head turned to one side; make sure he is not slumped, or curled up. Ask the nurses to help you if you would like some support.

4 Tuck him inside your clothes and hold him there, as if he were a baby kangaroo in a mother kangaroo's pouch.

The best position for you to be in while holding him like this, especially at first, is sitting down and leaning slightly back, perhaps with your feet up, so that he rests easily on you. You could perhaps put a blanket around him, over your clothes, to help hold him in place.

Held in skin-to-skin contact with her mother, as close as she can possibly be, Gabrielle is comfortable and content.

baby; and the medical staff are confident about supporting you in doing this.

Those NICUs that can help you give your baby kangaroo care will normally be happy for this to begin at around 30 weeks. Some units have staff who are very practiced and confident in this area, and are happy to begin even earlier: neonatal staff who are experienced in encouraging kangaroo care say that you can safely "kangaroo" a baby as tiny as 1 pound 6 ounces (600g).

If your baby is very premature or very small he is probably being monitored and tube-fed, and he may have CPAP (see page 30) too. This means he will be attached to some lead wires and tubes, so you will have to sit or recline near the equipment and not move around much. If your baby is older or more mature and does not need close monitoring, you can move around carefully, holding him tucked down your front. Many parents like to lie back on a sofa, a bed or in an armchair or rocking chair with their feet up.

How kangaroo care helps your baby

One question many parents ask about kangaroo care is how something so simple, natural and low-tech can make such a difference to the health of a premature baby. There are several good medical reasons why, but perhaps the simple answer is that babies like it. They are comfortable in the warmth, closeness, peace and security of being held close to their mother or father. Likely it reminds them of the safety of the uterus they left too early.

What is clear is that their health improves tremendously. There has been an immense amount of international research backing up the benefits of kangaroo care, from the UK, the US, Scandinavia, Germany and France, to India and Central and South America. UNICEF and The World Health Organization also recommend it.

Premature babies sleep better and breathe more easily when they are being "kangaroo'd." They cry and fidget less and, being calmer, they grow better. If babies have regular kangaroo care, they also breastfeed more easily, and their mothers can keep making milk for longer.

medically stable means still ill but holding steady and not getting any worse.

Kangaroo'd babies have fewer apnea (stop-breathing) and bradycardia (slowed heartbeat) attacks, and fewer body-temperature fluctuations—they stay warm, thanks to the warmth of your body. They develop fewer infections, leave their incubators sooner, and go home earlier.

Benefits for parents

Kangaroo care can be immensely comforting and calming for parents. Touching skin-to-skin and relaxing, without the artificial barriers of the incubator and any medical equipment, it is easier for you to bond with your baby.

MASSAGE

Massage can be a gentle way to show your love and care for your premature baby, and to soothe and comfort him. It also has proven health benefits, and many NICUs encourage mothers and fathers to massage their premature babies if the infants can cope with it. Research suggests it can have many positive effects, including improving digestion, helping babies sleep more soundly and deeply, encouraging them to breathe more easily, raising the levels of oxygen in their bloodstream, steadying their heart rate and even helping them gain weight more quickly.

Is your baby ready to be massaged?

Premature babies can be highly sensitive to touch. The more premature or unwell they are, the more hypersensitive they tend to be. Because of this, your baby may not be able to cope with a massage just yet. In some cases, unless the unit's neonatal nurses are trained in massaging premature babies, it may not be possible to give your child his first "proper" massage until he is nearly ready to go home. A very little gentle stroking or holding may be suggested instead.

When your baby has a small massage, you should not see his need for oxygen increase any more than it would when you change his diaper. After the massage, his level of oxygen saturation (the amount of oxygen in his blood) should go back to "resting level" or even increase slightly. If his oxygen saturation level drops or goes up sharply, this is a sign of stress, and would suggest that he is not able to cope

Ready for massage

Generally, a premature baby can be gently massaged on his back if he:

⋆ Is medically stable (see below). This is very important, because any touch for a premature baby who is still medically unstable can be distressing for him.

⋆ Is at least 28 weeks corrected age (see page 156), or four to six weeks old.

⋆ Is able to cope with having his diaper changed by his mother and father.

⋆ Is able to keep his own temperature fairly steady.

⋆ Has no lines or tubes that prevent him from being turned over on his stomach.

⋆ Does not need tube-feeding (see page 116).

You may even be able to massage your baby if he is on a ventilator because he has a long-term condition, such as BPD, but is otherwise medically stable.

A gentle massage for a premature baby

1 Undo your baby's clothing to waist level.

2 Dab some cotton wool in the oil and gently smooth a little on your baby's back.

3 Place your hands over your baby's back, but not touching him. Pause so he gets used to your hands being there.

4 Very slowly, gently massage his back with your right hand, your left hand lying gently on the back of his neck. Using just two fingertips, massage in small circles down by one side of your baby's spine (without touching the spine itself) and back up the other side.

5 Repeat using bigger circles (with more oil if needed).

6 Make the circles bigger still, going from the baby's back around to his abdomen.

7 To end, wipe off the excess oil with cotton, stroke his back gently, then pause for a moment with your hands just above his back.

8 Cover him gently with a blanket for the moment, rather than disturbing him by dressing him again.

After a massage

Afterward, it is a good idea to hang a notice on the end of his incubator, saying something like: *"Just had a massage. Please do not disturb."* Write the time at the end of it, so the nurses know how long to leave him resting.

with a massage yet. NICU staff may also advise that you do not give your baby a massage if he is having a bit of an "off" day—perhaps is having more spells of apnea or bradycardia than is normal for him, is more lethargic than usual or has been handled a lot that day already for tests or x-rays.

Every baby is highly individual. If you are not too sure about whether your baby is ready for a brief, light massage, talk about it to the nurse who knows him best, or the pediatrician or neonatologist. Keep a close eye on your baby's signals (see page 86) and use your own instincts as a parent to check that he is coping each time you give him even a small massage. If you are not sure whether he is ready just yet, perhaps it might be better to try some therapeutic touch or containment care (see page 98) to soothe him, until he is stronger and his nervous system is more mature.

How to massage your premature baby

There are different schools of thought about the "best" way to massage a premature baby. You may be in an NICU that has its own particular way of using massage or touch, which they could teach you and help you with. However, for most parents, a formula approach is not really what massaging their baby is about, and it is not the massage technique itself that is important. What matters most is your finding a safe way of enjoying loving contact with your baby.

Try to do your baby's massage at roughly the same time each day, and pick a quiet time. A good time is when there are no daily rounds going on, he is not hungry and he has not had anything done to him which may have upset and tired him (such as a blood test, tube suctions, a diaper change or a wash). Get everything ready first: some cotton wool, a little oil in a container standing in warm water and perhaps some music he likes (anything you know he can relax with).

Use plain vegetable oil. Never use aromatherapy oils on a premature baby's skin: they are too strong even when diluted down by a carrier oil. Do not use commercial baby oils, either, as they are mineral-based.

During the massage, always leave part of one hand or a fingertip on your baby, so that you never completely stop touching him. If you want to cover part of him up a little more, or dip the cotton wool into a bit more warm oil, keep, the back of one of your hands in contact with him as you do so.

How often you can massage depends on how well, or how fragile, your baby is at the moment. Many parents say they began with two or three times a week, working up to once a day if their baby liked it and could cope. Neonatal staff advise not mixing kangaroo care, cuddles and a massage all in the same day unless you can see from your baby's signals that he can definitely manage all this.

If there is a nurse at your NICU who knows about premature baby massage, you may like to get her to show you the first time, do the massage with her the second, and do it by yourself the third time, with her watching or helping. If not, you could ask the nurse who knows your baby best if she could support and help you to try the simple massage on page 108, and see if your baby likes it.

Hindered by tubes and monitors, contact is limited to Mom's finger in Marina's tiny hand.

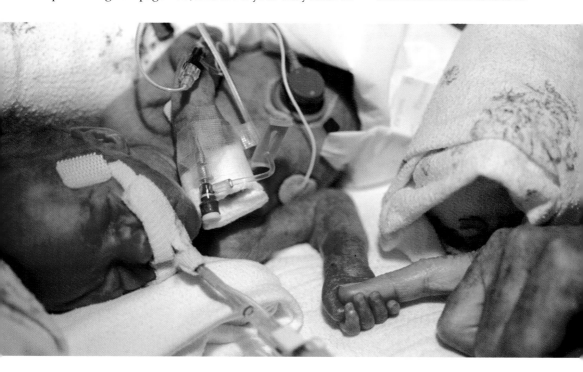

Playing with your premature baby

NICU nursing staff suggest that there are three important things to remember:

1 Find the right time.

2 Only do one thing at a time.

3 Be guided by your baby's own signals (see page 86).

Premature baby massage guidelines are there to help parents find out and learn about ways of touching their baby which are enjoyable (for both parties) and safe. It is very important to watch your baby's reactions: be guided by them, more than anything else. Is there anything special he seems to like? Or not like? Does he seem relaxed when you massage him? How does your baby let you know when he has had enough?

Back to sleep

It is fine to leave your baby sleeping on his front after a massage when he is in the NICU and attached to monitors that can tell you whether he is breathing well or not, and whether his heart rate is regular. At home, however, it is safest to turn your baby gently onto his back after 15 minutes or so, before you let him carry on sleeping.

If your baby cries

Try not to feel too discouraged if your baby cries the first time he has a massage, and maybe even the second or third time too. This may be because most of the touching he has had up until now has not been very pleasant. In fact, most of his experience of touch may have been uncomfortable or even painful. If a baby is usually only touched for diaper changing, blood sampling from his heel, being medically examined, having his IV lines or feeding tubes changed, it is not surprising that he may associate touch with something bad happening to him. But if you massage your baby regularly, he will come instead to associate your type of gentle touch or massage with pleasure and reassurance.

PLAYING WITH YOUR PREMATURE BABY

This may not be "playing" in the sense you would use with an older baby. It is play, however, if play is defined as something that catches and holds your baby's interest, and that he can join in with. Your premature baby may be able to cope with a little (a very little) of this type of interaction at as young as 33 or 34 weeks. But how much he will be able to manage depends on many different things, including how well or unwell he is, what medical problems he has had, and how he has been nursed and generally cared for. It is also dependent upon whether or not your baby has any particular medical condition that means he might find this sort of interaction especially tiring or difficult to deal with.

You will not necessarily need bright rattles or soft cuddly toys, though you might like to try showing them to your baby, perhaps just placing them in his incubator, to see if he is interested. You can try putting a brightly colored toy within his sight line but where he can easily move his gaze away if he does not want to look at it. However, he will probably be more interested in your face, touch and voice, and these will bring him comfort and help him relax and be calm. Play will come as your baby gets better and grows and develops.

Even though he needs a nasal cannula to help him breathe, he can still enjoy being bathed by his mother.

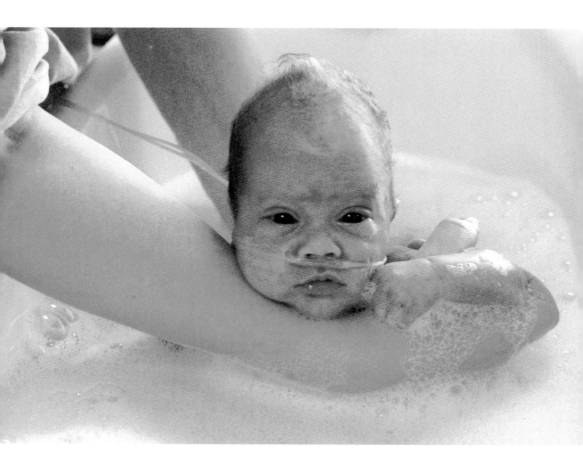

A premature baby's food will contain:

★ more calories for energy, as a premature baby can use up a great deal, especially if he is stressed or unwell

★ more fat, since he needs this for energy but will not have much of his own stored up yet

★ more protein, which is very important for growing

★ more water, because premature babies can become dehydrated very quickly and their water intake needs to be carefully and individually monitored

★ more vitamins and minerals, because a baby usually builds up his stores in the last 12 weeks he spends in his mother's uterus; the earlier your baby was born, the lower his store of vital minerals and vitamins will be

How long to play

The awake time for a premature baby aged 33–34 weeks can vary greatly depending on many different factors—the same ones that determine how ready he is for play. Even if he is well, however, and has been cared for very sensitively and protectively, you will probably find that he can only cope with very brief periods of interaction or concentration: perhaps a couple of minutes at the most. This may not sound like much. Yet if you think that if your baby had not been born early he would never have felt the touch of a hand, or even looked at anything, for several weeks yet, it may begin to seem like a good deal.

So long as your baby is well and stable, a good time to try interacting with him is when he is rested, calm and awake of his own accord—that is, has not been woken up by someone else. Find out if there are any regular times when he is awake and time play for one of these. If there are no regular times yet, just sit quietly by him (perhaps reading or resting) until he is awake and seems alert.

At 34 weeks, premature babies can usually only cope with one thing at a time. Your baby may enjoy touch, listening, and looking. But dealing with all three (or even two) forms of stimulation at once is usually too much.

Try to observe your baby while you are "playing" with him. He is telling you how he feels with his body language, the expression on his face, the way he is holding his hands or arms, his muscle tension, the rate of his breathing and his heart rate, even the color tone of his skin. Does he seem to be coping with the contact, and enjoying it? Or do you feel that perhaps now is not such a good time? Be guided by your baby's signals and try to trust your own instincts as a parent too—they are usually right.

Touching

Try holding or stroking him softly along his hand or feet, one at a time, or his back. If your baby can cope with this, try feeling his arms and legs, gently but not with a ticklish feathery-light touch—babies do not seem to like that. If he does not seem comfortable with this, leave it and try again another time. There may be other forms of touching that your own baby especially likes. Some premature babies find a hand cupping the head soothing. Others like their feet being held, or their shoulders supported by an adult's hand. If your baby is well enough for a bath, you may well find that he loves being held securely in the gently moving water.

Looking

Let your baby see your face about 8–10 inches (20–25cm) away. Smile or just look at him calmly and "speak" with your eyes. Allow him to focus on your face. Then slowly move your head from side to side. Watch to see if his eyes follow you. You may notice that even just half a minute of this may be enough. If your baby seems ready and interested in interacting with you in this way, even for short periods, the play-looking can help him to develop and coordinate his sight.

Ella needs to be fed through a nasogastric tube, but, touching her own face with one hand and holding tight to her mother's finger with the other, show that she is serene and relaxed.

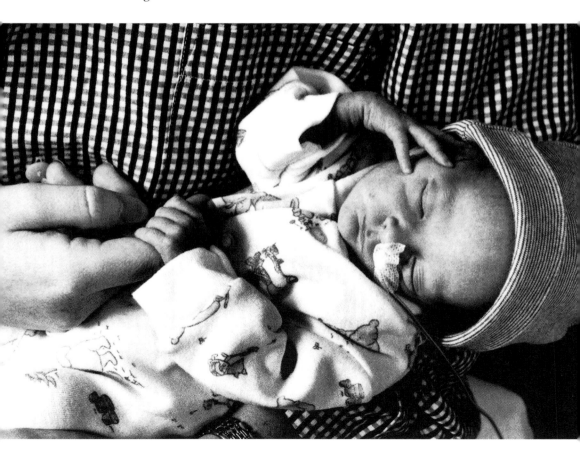

Methods of tube-feeding

At the very beginning, the milk may be dripped gently down the tube all the time. This is called *continuous feeding*.

The next stage is hourly feeds, then two-hourly, then every three hours, as your baby is gradually able to cope with larger and larger amounts of milk at a time. This sort of small, regular meal of milk is called a *bolus*.

Talking

Talk softly to your baby, recite nursery rhymes, poetry—anything you feel comfortable saying to him and that you feel he might like to listen to. If you begin to see signals that you know mean your baby would prefer just to be peaceful for now without any stimulation, leave it for a while and try again later.

FEEDING YOUR PREMATURE BABY

Feeding a premature baby can at first look like a difficult and specialized job that only the nurses can do, especially if the baby is very premature, fragile or unwell. But it isn't.

If you would like to be properly involved in feeding your own baby and have enough time to do it, you can. In fact, you are probably the best person in the world to do it. Some NICUs are 100 percent behind parents who want to feed their own babies, others are less enthusiastic. However, with the staff's support, parents can help with all the different premature baby feeding methods, including tube-feeds.

Either the mother or father (or both) can take over the responsibility for tube-feeding, bottle-feeding, cup-feeding and (if you are the mother) eventually breastfeeding your baby. Depending on how much time you can spend at the NICU, you can do this part-time—so that a certain feeding time or times are saved for you when you can come into the unit—or almost full-time, if you are able to be around most of the time. Either way you'll need to go home for a few hours each night to get some sleep.

Mothers can also do something else very special for their babies that no one else can—give them their expressed breast milk. This is probably the single most important thing you can do to help your baby grow strong and well. Even if you only make a little bit, it will still be very valuable for your baby, and it can be topped up with formula. However, if you find you cannot express your milk, you can still be fully involved in your own baby's care by using a tube, cup or bottle to give him a special premature-baby formula instead.

What babies need

Premature babies want feeding and nourishing just like other babies. It is just that they need to be fed in different ways until they are able to coordinate their sucking, swallowing and breathing to take their milk from the breast, or from a bottle, for themselves. (They can often suck on your finger or a pacifier quite strongly long before they can breast- or bottle-feed.) They also need a special milk mixture until their digestive systems and kidneys reach the "term baby" stage.

IV feeding

IV (intravenous) feeding involves giving special liquid food by way of a fine tube, into a vein. At first the liquid food will be a mixture of sugar (glucose), salts and water; later some amino acids (protein building blocks), plus some fats and minerals may be added. IV feeding is used

A nurse feeds a baby through a nasogastric tube.

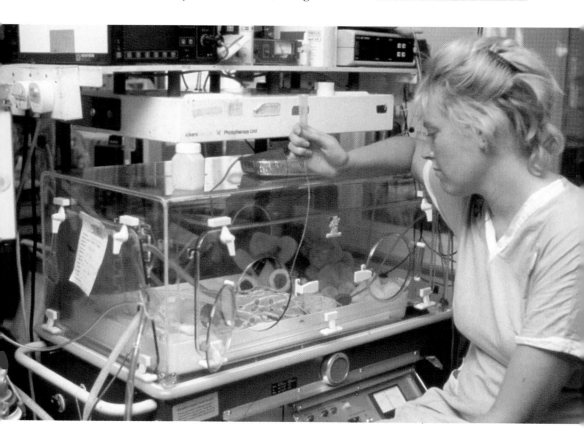

"I couldn't wait for the day when I could first hold Annie on my lap and cup-feed her myself. But I was so scared of pulling out a monitor wire or a tube that when the nurse put her in my arms and encouraged me to feed her I just sat there rigid. It was a relief to put her back and I was so upset I cried buckets afterwards. Yet three weeks later I hardly noticed all the wires and was getting her in and out to feed her all the time on my own, just like a nurse would."

Jo, Annie's mother

Cup-feeding and breastfeeding

Babies who cup-feed are more likely to be able to breastfeed than babies who don't. As soon as your baby is old enough to lick from a cup he can also lick from you, and you can begin to help him get used to the fact that your breast means food and comfort. This is the beginning of being able to breastfeed.

1 Try to get your baby to lick a little expressed milk off your nipple.

2 When he has got used to this, try expressing a little into his mouth as he nuzzles at your breast.

3 The final stage is helping him latch onto your breast with his mouth so he can try to suckle for himself.

when a baby is too premature (from 23 to 28 weeks), too small (under 2 pounds 3 ounces/1000g) or too unwell to digest milk. It may be given for the first few hours or even first few days after birth, depending on how prematurely the baby was born and also on how well or unwell he is.

So long as the baby is well and stable enough, even while he is being fed intravenously he may also be able to cope with beginning to learn to enjoy licking milk from his mother's nipple as a preliminary to breastfeeding.

Tube-feeding

This method feeds milk through a fine plastic tube, and is used when your baby's digestive system is ready for food by mouth but he cannot yet suck and drink properly, for himself. The tube usually threads down via the baby's nose or mouth, then into his stomach and is known as a naso- or orogastric tube. There is also another sort of feeding tube that goes straight through the stomach and down into the small intestine. This is called a transpyloric tube. It gives small amounts of milk continuously, and might be used if a baby is very small. Your baby's food may be formula milk, breast milk or a mixture of both.

Your baby may be fed by tube alone for several days, for a few weeks or even for a few months—just how long depends on how well he is, and how prematurely he was born. As he becomes more mature and stronger, he can be introduced to cup-feeding, breastfeeding or bottle-feeding gradually, while still having top-up feedings by tube.

You can give your baby small amounts of your breast milk down this tube from the very beginning. It is also possible to introduce him to the idea of breastfeeding while he is still tube-feeding, just as soon as he can lick milk off your nipple.

Many NICUs will encourage a mother to hold her baby against her partly bared breast just before a tube-feed when the baby is becoming hungry, then to express a little milk onto her nipple and areola, and position her baby's face so that he can both smell the milk and reach the nipple. If a baby is ready he will often begin to try to lick the milk off. The lovely smell and taste of it, plus the special scent of the mother's skin, can all set the scene to help him begin to try some practice sucking, a first important step towards learning to breastfeed.

Practice sucking

If your baby is able to do a little practice sucking every time he has a tube-feed, this is very good for him. Research suggests it helps babies' digestion, so they tend to put on weight faster, and helps coordinate their breathing-sucking-swallowing, so they can go on to cup-feeding or breastfeeding more quickly. It is best if he can practice sucking on your nipple, but many units also use a pacifier.

Positioning your baby in the right way for practice sucking at your breast is very important, and a tiny shift of position can make a huge difference to whether your baby is able to try suckling or not. Hold a baby in one way and it all seems perfectly easy, hold him slightly differently and he is not happy or comfortable so he either won't try, or he won't be able to and will get discouraged very quickly.

Try asking the staff to help you if you are not too sure, as often as you need to, since most will be only too glad to support you. If your baby still has a nose tube taped in place, try to hold him so that the tube-free nostril is facing away from your nipple so that he can breathe. If he has a tube passing down into his mouth, make sure that it is taped at the side of his mouth and cheek rather than down over his bottom lip and chin.

Cup-feeding

With cup-feeding, you hold your baby cuddled comfortably upright on your lap, and gently lift a small cup of milk (like a little medicine cup with rounded edges) to his mouth, tilting it very slightly so a tiny bit goes against his lips. The fact that the milk is against his lips rather than poured into his mouth means that the baby himself is in control of his own drinking, and that he is less likely to choke or become stressed by the fear of choking. Some nurses also suggest swaddling the baby so that he cannot knock the cup with his hands.

Your baby will be able to smell and taste the milk, which he cannot do when he is tube-fed, and because it

"One reason given to parents for not cup-feeding is that it could be dangerous because a baby might breathe in the milk. However, this simply isn't true. I think if there had been a single case of this happening... I would have heard about it."

Sandra Lang, cup-feeding pioneer and Infant Feeding Consultant to the World Health Organization and UNICEF

"I really did try, I stuck at it for eight days. It seemed like forever and I could hardly get any milk out. It was really winding me up. I couldn't believe something so natural was so difficult, and I felt miserable and stupid because it was like—my body couldn't stay pregnant for long enough and now even my boobs didn't work... So he was fed on formula and he's fine. Getting bigger every day."

Cherie, Cole's mother

Try to feed him when he's not tired

Does your baby seem to be tired out by having his diaper changed, being dressed, examined by the doctors, having his heel prick tests? If so, try to feed him before any of this is done, or some time afterward, so he has a chance to recover. Check when any routine tests or procedures will be done and ask the nurses to help you work out a feeding plan timed to avoid these interventions. Suckling takes energy and if he is tired, he will not be able to feed very well.

Jacky attempts to breastfeed Marina, born at 24 weeks.

smells and tastes good this encourages him to try to drink for himself. Within a few days or a week or so he will catch on to the idea and begin first to lick from the cup, then lap at it like a kitten. Later, he will progress to sipping the milk. The next step is to give him a bottle or try breastfeeding, if you would like to.

Many mothers like to hold their baby against their naked skin, perhaps partly undoing their blouse or lifting their T-shirt, so he can smell their special scent, especially if they are feeding their baby their own breast milk, and/or planning to try and breastfeed fully later on. Skin-to-skin contact like this, or kangaroo care (see page 105), also helps your body produce breast milk.

A premature baby will probably need a combination of tube-feeding and cup-feeding for several weeks, gradually learning to take more milk from the cup each time, then perhaps having one whole feeding from a cup, then two… and so on until he takes most or all of his milk like this. (You can continue until your baby is ready to take all his food either by breastfeeding or bottle-feeding.) You need not worry about how much milk he drinks this way at first. His nurse will be able to work out if he needs a top-up by tube, and if so, how much extra he needs each time.

If your NICU does not cup-feed their babies If you are interested in feeding your baby this way but the unit does not offer it, one possible gentle way into a discussion with your baby's nurses is to mention that you have been reading about cup-feeding (perhaps even show them this small section here). Say that you have heard it can triple the rate of successful breastfeeding, which it can. Ask them what their own thoughts are on this. If they seem interested, ask if they might possibly like to talk to staff on a unit that does cup-feed about helping you to do this. The senior staff there would probably be very glad to talk to nurses from your unit—as one professional to another— about their own experience of it. There is also a book about cup-feeding aimed at nursing professionals which they might find interesting (see *References*).

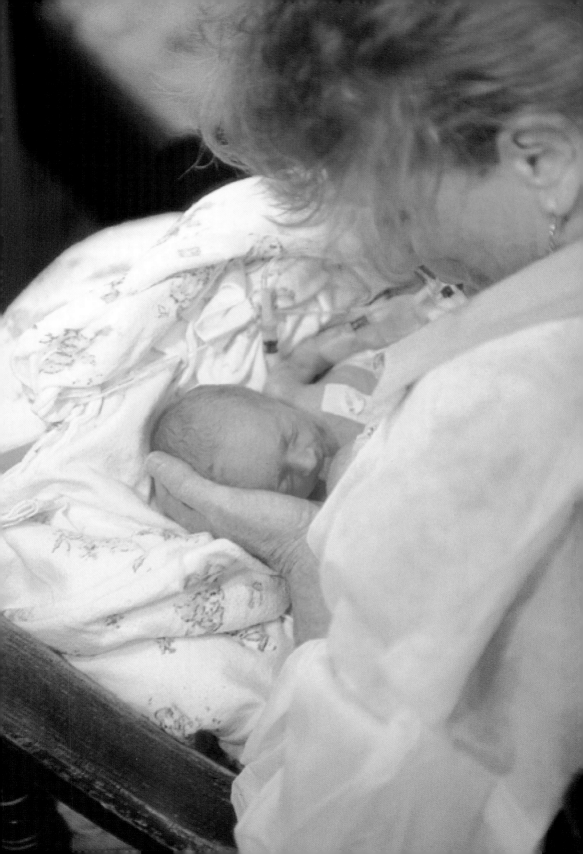

"I had always wanted to feed him myself, I had decided right back when I was only a few weeks pregnant I would breastfeed my baby. But I had an emergency caesarean at 29 weeks, and he was so ill at first. I felt bad for several days afterwards, then I was too upset about Michael being in intensive care to really get any expressing going. I just couldn't face it, on top of everything else."

Kate, Michael's mother

If you would like to breast-feed your premature baby, it is usually better to, not to bottle-feed at all, if possible. This is because babies suckle on bottle nipples in one way and breast nipples in another. Trying to learn both at once may confuse and stress your baby, and he may not be able to breastfeed after all. Instead, cup-feeding, which uses a different mouth action on your baby's part, can be a good halfway house between tube-feeding and breastfeeding.

Bottle-feeding

Once a premature baby is mature enough to manage sucking, swallowing and breathing at the same time, you can begin to feed him using a specially made small bottle which only holds 1–2oz (25–50ml) milk and a special nipple that is as small, soft and flexible as possible. There are many different designs and you may find your baby likes one better than another.

The bottle will contain a powdered milk formula mixture that is designed specifically for preterm babies. Because his digestive system and organs such as the kidneys and the liver are not mature yet, and because he may be unwell, a premature baby will need a very particular formula mixture customized just for him. Your baby's personal milk mixture may need to be changed and adapted as he grows and matures, and the dietician, pediatrician or neonatologist will follow your baby's progress carefully to suggest changes in the formula mix as and when needed.

Bottle-feeding will help your baby flourish and grow, and you may find that it is the best way for you and your child. Many mothers of premature babies—even those who have successfully breastfed their other children—find that they cannot breastfeed. This may be because they are often very tired, stressed, not well, have not had the support needed to breastfeed or simply cannot make enough milk for their premature baby's needs. Some mothers may have other heavy commitments such as a home and other children to care for, have had to return to work, or live a long way away from the unit, which means they are not able to spend long hours at the NICU each day.

Gently preparing your baby In his early weeks of life, it's possible that most of the things happening to a sick, premature baby in or around his mouth have been unpleasant, maybe even painful—endotracheal tubes, feeding tubes, nasal tubes taped and re-taped to his cheeks. Yet you can make sure you offer some gentle touches around your baby's mouth, to help show him that touches in and around his mouth can feel good too. For instance, research suggests that gentle, loving stroking of your baby's lips and around his mouth can make for easier feeding. Offering your baby chances for comfort-sucking can also help. Signs that your baby might like to comfort-suck include trying to bring his hands up to his mouth, turning his head and opening his mouth, and making little sucking movements.

Positioning your baby so both of you are comfortable
Hold him with his head slightly raised, close to the warmth of your body, perhaps with his head and upper body against a bared patch of your skin so he can smell and feel you. Ask the nurses to help you here if you are not sure if the position is quite right. A bit of privacy can help create a small oasis of peace and quiet for you both to enjoy the cuddling, closeness, and one-to-one time of the bottle-feed, so if the NICU is busy, you could ask for screens to be placed around you for a while.

Taking it at your baby's own pace Try to take your time, and let your baby set the pace of the feeding. You don't need to hurry it along by wiggling the nipple in your baby's mouth or prodding him gently awake to encourage him to take more or drink a little faster. If he stops sucking, let him rest for a while.

Bottle-feeding can sometimes be a little trickier than breast- or cup-feeding because the milk can flow faster. Prodding the baby, or moving the bottle about, twisting/turning it to get him to take more milk may look like an effective way to get your baby to take in more food and certainly, in the old days, neonatal units took quite a lot of pride in using these methods to make sure babies drank the "required" amount of milk every time. But most now know that forcing milk down, without the baby drinking it himself, can make feeding stressful for a baby and may cause apnea and bradycardia attacks.

Try not to be discouraged if, initially, it seems that the nurses can get your baby to feed more than you can. This often happens, perhaps because parents cuddle their baby so gently and lovingly, that, feeling safe and secure, he responds by falling happily asleep. Sitting a baby up and

"It was the one thing I felt I could give her that no one else could. And watching her grow and get better on my milk—that was so good."

Claudie, Luis's mother

Giving your baby your own breast milk doesn't mean you have to struggle to give him a hearty 20-minute breastfeed each mealtime. He may only need a couple of teaspoons at a time to get some of the very special benefits.

Breast milk for premature babies

Research shows that the breast milk mothers make for their premature babies is different from the milk that mothers make when their babies are born at term. And the milk slowly changes too, to cater for a premature baby's changing needs as he or she becomes bigger, stronger and more mature.

Are pacifiers okay?

Some premature-baby feeding experts believe that if you are planning to breastfeed your baby or are already doing so, he should not usually be given a pacifier. This is because a baby sucks on a pacifier or bottle nipple in very different ways than on his mother's nipples. So if he practices sucking on a pacifier, he may not be able to breast-fee.

However, once he is upset, a premature baby finds it difficult to calm himself and he uses up much-needed calories crying. Sometimes, if a baby is very unsettled, and other comforting methods are not working (see page 100), having a pacifier to suck on can be really helpful.

gently "burping" him can wake him up a little. So can touching the soles of his feet, making eye contact with him or talking to him. It may be, however, that what your baby is "saying" is that he is just not ready at that point to take a whole bottle, but he is ready for a cuddle.

Most NICUs usually suggest 20–30 minutes for a feeding, depending on the baby, so as not to tire him right out. If a feeding goes on for more than half an hour, it can leave a baby exhausted. Be guided by your own baby's signals—those, and your own special instincts as a parent, will let you know better than anything else whether he would like to carry on feeding or stop for now.

Can I breastfeed as well? A mother's own milk supply usually drops slowly over time if she does bottle-feed. This is because the more stimulation your breasts have, either from a baby's sucking or from expressing, the more milk you will make. The reverse is also true: the less expressing or sucking you receive, the less milk you make.

Breastfeeding

Breast milk can do many things for your baby that formula milk cannot. It is not just a food—it is a powerful medicine too because it can protect against infections, help your baby's digestion so he puts on weight more easily, encourages his brain development and much, much more. You do not need very much of it at first either—just a few regular drops can do your baby a lot of good. If you can possibly give even a little you are doing a lot more than just feeding your baby. You will be providing an important part of his medical treatment as well.

Scientists have found over a hundred different good things in breast milk—proteins, enzymes, antibodies and other ingredients that will help protect your baby against illnesses and infections. This is particularly important for premature babies because their immune systems are not yet strong or mature enough to fight off germs very well.

If your baby is too young, too immature, or too unwell to nurse, and you are finding you can only manage to express a few drops of milk into a container—that's fine. A 2 pound (900g) baby, for example, may only be needing one and a half teaspoons of milk an hour anyway, given via a tube. If you make less than this, it can be added into some formula. Even very small amounts of your milk can do your baby a lot of good.

Overcoming difficulties Feeding your baby on your own breast milk in an often stressful, artificial environment like the NICU can be hard. Whether you manage to breastfeed or not depends partly on how determined you yourself are, and on how much time you have. It also depends on how much help and support you have from the staff there.

You may not be very well yourself after your baby's birth. By the time you are feeling a bit better, it is harder for your body to start making enough milk to feed your baby. You are in an unnatural, high-tech environment and you may be very stressed if your baby is not well.

Breastfeeding may be natural but that does not mean it is instantly easy or instinctive, even for mothers of healthy term babies. Only some 65 percent of them try breastfeeding and only around four in ten are still breastfeeding when their babies are six weeks old. And mothers of term babies have something that really helps get breastfeeding going—a healthy baby regularly sucking at the breast; most mothers of premature babies do not.

On just about every front, mothers of premature babies have a great deal more to cope with than do mothers of healthy term babies. Yet skilled and sympathetic help from the unit staff can make a huge difference. A study in Britain revealed that the average number of NICU mothers who went home with their premature babies breastfeeding was between one and two in ten, yet in the NICUs that went all out to help mothers nurse, it was nearer to eight out of every ten. If you feel you are not getting enough help to try breastfeeding, seek help outside the NICU (see Helplines, page 203).

Lastly, establishing breastfeeding can be a matter of time. How much can you spend on getting your milk supply going and keeping it going as you shuttle to and from the NICU? You may have other young children to care for and the hospital may be a long way from where

Expressing by pump

Get ready in the same way as you would to express by hand. Sometimes it helps to begin expressing a bit gently by hand first, to encourage your milk to flow. Pump until your milk stops flowing.

"Pump, pump, pump—they were constantly on at me to keep using it. I could only get out a few drops each time. It was like being a cow on a milking machine, it was so undignified. We got this little bit each day. The nurses gave Susie that down the tube and said it really was much better for her than none."

Marine, Susie's mother

The more often you express your milk, the more you will make

Try to express 8 to 10 times a day: some mothers have found it helps to set their watches to remind them.

You can have about five hours unbroken sleep at night without diminishing your milk supply. However, it is very important to try to express at least once during the night.

Added extras

If your baby needs anything special or extra—perhaps more iron if he is short of it, or more calories if he has been losing weight, or more water if he is becoming dehydrated—the staff at the NICU would, with your permission, add whatever extra is needed to your breast milk.

Spending quiet time together in the darkened NICU

you live. Finding the time and peace to make breast milk for your baby can be hard.

Expressing your breast milk Expressing is the best way of getting your milk supply up and running—and keeping it going—until your baby is ready to breastfeed. There are many different ways to do this, and mothers usually find that there is one particular method that suits them best.

There are several slightly different "by hand" methods, small plastic handheld pumps, some of which can be discreetly used with a shawl or big scarf draped over your shoulder, and electric breast pumps which the hospital will have available for you to use, usually in a quiet private room. You may also be able to rent or borrow one to use at home. Some electric pumps are designed so you can pump both your breasts at once, which can save a good deal of

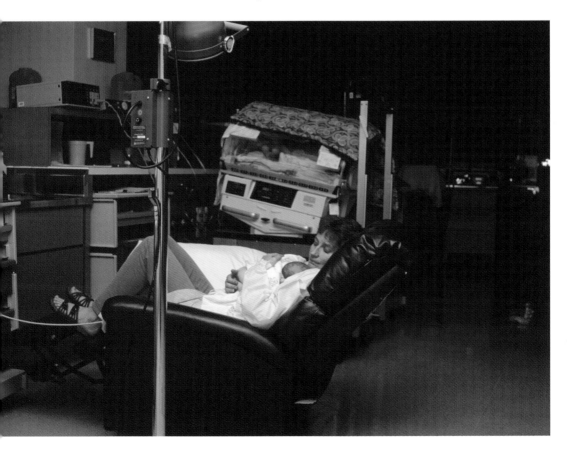

time. Electric pumps can be very quick and efficient, but many mothers also say that they can be uncomfortable, as their suction is pretty strong. Some mothers find that they like to use the breast pump for a couple of minutes after they have hand-expressed, as this can release any milk that had been left behind more efficiently.

The hospital's lactation consultant, or one of the nurses, should be able to sit with you as often as you need them to and show you how to express your milk. According to breastfeeding specialists, it works best if you begin trying to express your milk within just six hours of your baby's birth, if you can. The sooner you begin, the easier it is; the longer you leave it, the harder it can be. It may not work too well the first time, or even the first few times, but it gets much easier the more often you do it.

If you have had a general anesthetic for an emergency Cesarean and are still feeling groggy, ask if the lactation consultant, or a nurse or midwife experienced in helping mothers breastfeed, can express your milk for you until you feel more able to start learning this gentle skill yourself. Even without a general anesthetic, Cesarean mothers need plenty of support, as the abdomen will be sore and they will need help in getting to a comfortable sitting position in bed.

If the staff do not seem really able to help you here, ask whether there is someone from an organization such as La Leche who comes into the unit (there often is). If there isn't anyone, call up one of the breastfeeding help organizations yourself (see Helplines, page 203) and ask if they have any counselors in your area who can come and see you, either at the NICU or in your own home if you are back there by now.

Helping your milk supply Perhaps for the first few weeks you may only be making a little breast milk. But as you get more and more used to expressing, you will produce more. Don't panic if the amount you are making sometimes drops. This is a completely normal reaction to being worried, tired or stressed. If your milk supply is falling, but you would like to keep it going, have a talk with your

Expressing by hand

1 Make sure you are warm and comfortable, and try to be relaxed. Wash your hands, and have a sterile container ready to catch your milk. Think about your baby, look at a picture of him, inhale his special scent from a piece of his clothing or blanket, or sit by him to encourage your milk to begin flowing.

2 Gently massage your breasts for a few minutes. If you are feeling tense or your shoulders are aching, ask someone to massage and knead your shoulders and upper back. Then massage your areola, the colored surrounding part of your nipple, with your thumb above and fingers below.

3 Now try moving your entire hand firmly inward, toward your chest. Press your fingers and thumb together and move your hand away again, gently squeezing out colostrum or milk. Try to move your hand around to empty out all the different parts of your breast.

4 If the flow slows down, try changing to the other breast. Go from one side to the other several times in one session.

5 If you are having any difficulty or are unsure of how you are doing, seek help from the hospital lactation specialist—that's what they are there for.

Breast milk storage

Always:

* Use a fresh, sterile container.

* Refrigerate milk within one hour after pumping.

* Use or freeze the milk within 48 hours.

* Use frozen milk within 2–3 months.

(From Health Canada. *Health Canada. Family-Centred Maternity and Newborn Care: National Guidelines*, Minister of Public Works and Government Services, Ottawa, 2000.)

hospital breastfeeding counselor (if there is one) or with a neonatal nurse or midwife who has a special interest in helping mothers breastfeed, or to a breastfeeding help organization. They will be able to advise you about the many things that you can do to increase your supply.

If gentle hand massage and expressing does not help you make more milk in the usual way, some units will offer a mother some medication called Metoclopramide. It is really an anti-nausea drug, but for many women it has a useful side effect—they find the amount of breast milk they produce doubles. It does not work for everyone, however, and while it seems to have no adverse side effects, not all doctors will prescribe it.

Making expressing easier Many mothers say it helps to place warm towels on their breasts or to massage their breasts in a warm bath as it relaxes them and helps the milk to flow, though this is easier to manage at home. Sitting next to your baby and looking at him, either with your back to the room or with some screens around you so you have a little privacy, helps too. It may help to have one hand on your baby (or as nearly touching his head or body as possible) and another working a small handheld breast pump. If you cannot sit next to your baby you may find it helps to be looking at a picture of him, or holding some clothes he has been wearing or a little blanket he has been using, and breathing in his own special scent from this. It is best to be somewhere nice and quiet: expressing milk when you are watching TV or talking to someone does not seem to work very well.

Enjoying a bottle-feed, and an opportunity for closeness

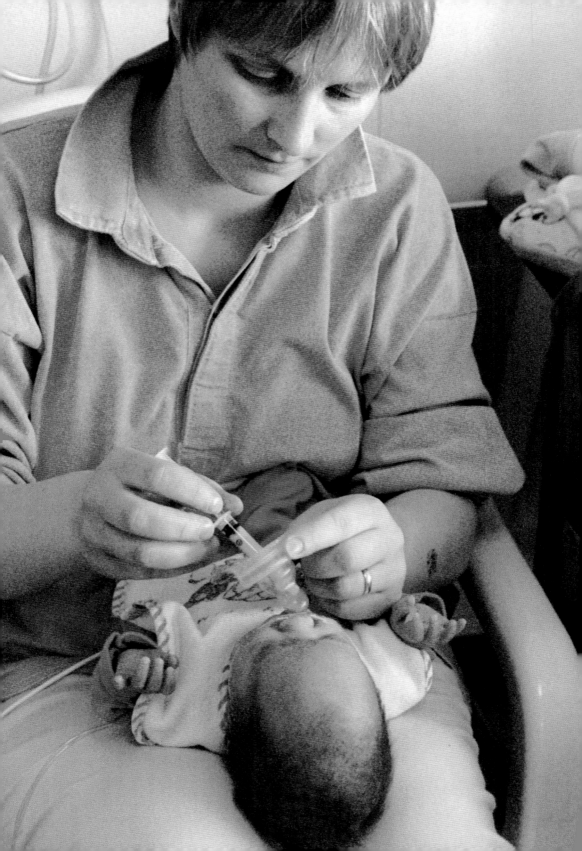

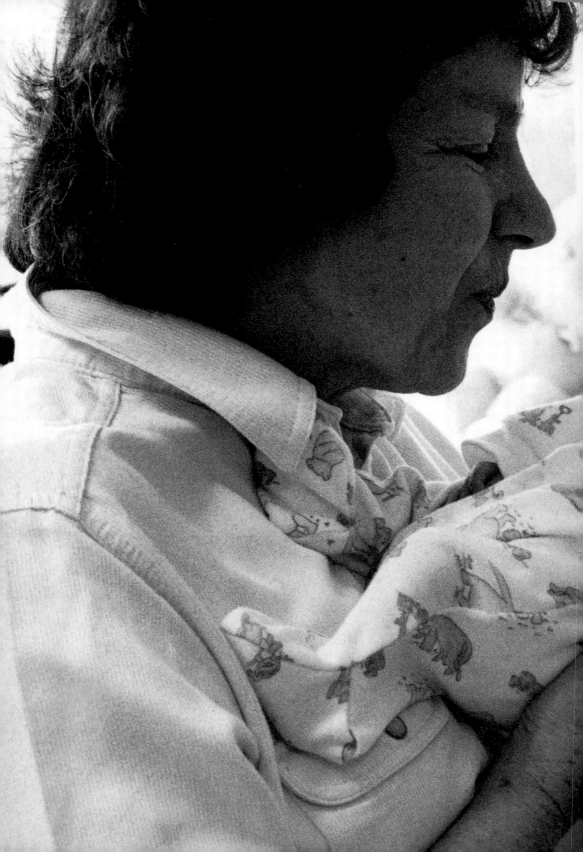

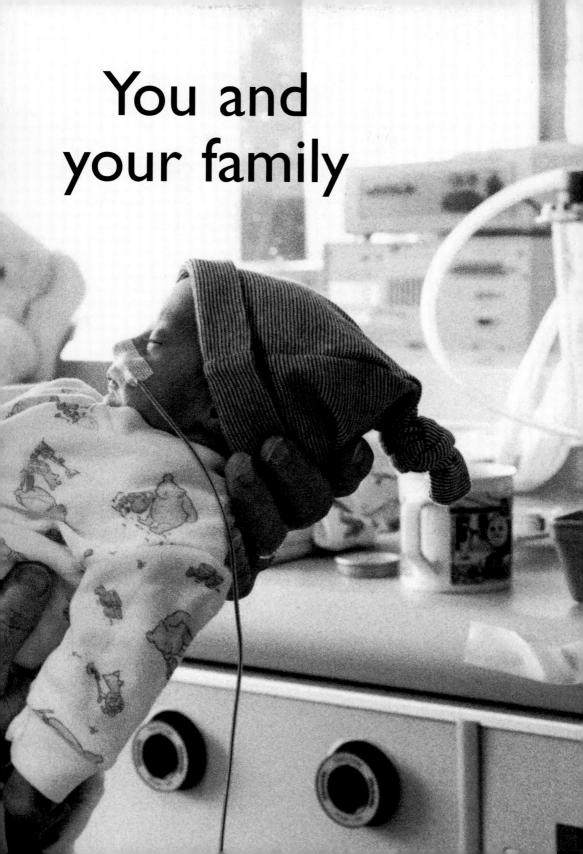

You and
your family

"I coped somehow while Jasmine was really ill, I think by just taking one day at a time. It was when she was virtually well out of intensive care for the last three weeks that I cracked. All the feelings I hadn't let myself feel finally hit me. I felt depressed, drained, angry, frustrated. And totally fed up. I had just suddenly had enough of all of it. I suppose I just hadn't had the space for all that before, I'd been too worried about her."

Gillie, mother of Jasmine, whose twin brother died

Having a premature baby brings challenges and stresses to the whole family. You probably expected to be home with your baby after a few days, not having to spend weeks or months almost living at the hospital. And, while you may have prepared your older children for the arrival of a new brother or sister, they probably didn't expect to meet her wired up to a bank of monitors, or that you would be spending so much time—away from them—in the NICU. But there are many things that can help you cope with this upheaval in your and your family's life.

WHAT ABOUT YOU?

As a mother, you may feel as though taking care of yourself is just too much to cope with, what with worrying about your baby and your other responsibilities. But, if you can possibly take some care of yourself, you will be in far better shape to help, care for and protect your baby and to look after your family. There are practical things you can do that only take a few minutes, and which could help your own energy levels and well-being greatly.

Getting your post-natal health care

New mothers of premature babies frequently miss out on ordinary medical post-partum help and care. For instance, if you have just had a baby, you would visit our doctor shortly after returning home. Unfortunately, this arrangement tends to fall apart if you are spending all of your time in the NICU.

One way of overcoming this is to ask for post-partum checks at the NICU. Many units, though by no means all, can arrange for your examinations—for example to see how any stitches from an episiotomy, tear or caesarean incision, are healing—to be carried out at the NICU or elsewhere in the hospital.

Soothing sore perineal stitches

Nearly half of all new mothers who have given birth vaginally need stitches to repair a perineal tear or an episiotomy. Perineal stitches should be feeling much better within ten days. If they aren't—and particularly if there is any redness or soreness—this is not something that is likely to get better on its own and needs medical attention. If you cannot see your own doctor, ask the nurse practitioner in the NICU if you can see a doctor or nurse practitioner on staff or if they can help you make an appointment quickly to see an obstetrician. There may be an infection, which can be healed with antibiotics, or the stitching may be too tight or have trapped a nerve, or there may be other problems that can all be sorted out by an expert.

Perineal stitches make sitting for long thoroughly uncomfortable. This is especially important for mothers of premature babies, who may find they are doing far more actual sitting because they are in the NICU watching over their babies, rather than moving around freely at home.

Dealing with back pain

Around six in ten new mothers have back pain in the days or even weeks after birth, and sitting for long periods on uncomfortable hospital chairs can make the pain worse. Some of the tips mentioned here can help, but if your back is really painful or seems to be getting worse, try to make an appointment to see a practitioner such as a massage therapist or physiotherapist who specializes in helping new mothers. You could feel so much better after even a single session that it will be worth making the time.

Once your doctor or midwife has given you permission to increase your physical activity, some gentle exercise—such as a relaxing swim in a nearby pool or a half-hour walk on a sunny day—can do much to bring welcome relief, as well as offer a boost to your spirits.

Depression and anxiety

Some feelings of depression and anxiety (often called "baby blues") are usual even for mothers of healthy babies born at term, and as the mother of a premature baby you have difficulties to cope with that term mothers do not have. Feelings of distress and anxiety are a completely normal and reasonable reaction to the sudden, traumatic birth of a premature baby who is sick, and may be in intensive care. They should start to fade as your baby grows stronger and you are able to become more involved with her care and more confident that she will be fine after all.

Making yourself more comfortable:

★ Always sit on a soft cushion.

★ Don't sit for too long at a time without a break.

★ Use the soft, old-fashioned, cotton sanitary napkins for protection rather than the new, thin, vinyl-coated, panty-liner type.

★ Wear roomy cotton briefs.

★ Find a bath you can use to have a daily warm, healing and antiseptic soak, in water with a big handful of salt added.

Relieving back pain:

★ Use a small squishy pillow underneath you or as support for your lower back.

★ Find something to prop your feet up about 5–8 inches (15–20cm).

★ Try not to sit for more than 30 minutes at a time: get up for a stretch or walk around for a moment or two, and try to do some gentle back stretching and strengthening exercises.

★ Stop muscles stiffening up and soothe discomfort with a hot water bottle, half-filled so it's pliable and can go around your lower back for about ten minutes.

Postpartum depression

★ If you have your baby prematurely you may be more likely to experience PPD.

★ PPD can start within the first few weeks of the baby's birth.

★ Symptoms include constant exhaustion but with difficulty in sleeping, feeling increasingly detached from everything around you, worrying obsessively about the baby even if she is getting better, weepiness, irritability and anxiety.

Find someone to talk to, for example:

★ your partner

★ a friend or relative

★ one of the nurses at the unit—anyone there you like and trust, such as your baby's "named" nurse (the one especially in charge of your baby's care)

★ your midwife

★ another parent on the unit

★ a parents' counselor or psychotherapist at the unit

★ a helpline, see page 203.

However, sometimes depression can last for many months and still be there long after your baby is well and back home with you. When this happens, doctors call it postpartum depression (PPD). Experts say that if PPD is recognized and treated properly and promptly you can be much better within as little as three months. Unrecognized and untreated it may persist for months, sometimes years.

Recognizing postpartum depression Suspect possible PPD if the way you feel is making it increasingly hard for you to cope with your daily life and/or if your baby is starting to thrive, but you are feeling steadily worse. Ask for help right away. Tell your obstetrician or doctor, or your midwife or one of the neonatal nurses on your baby's ward whom you like and trust, a parents' counselor or breastfeeding counselor, or call one of the groups on page 203 that assist new mothers with postpartum depression.

Treatment All forms of PPD are treatable, and in many cases with the right help you will be feeling much better within a few short weeks. The two main strands of treatment are counseling and medication. The latter can include hormone treatment (sometimes with estrogen, sometimes progesterone, sometime thyroid hormone), mild antidepressants, which are not addictive, and tranquilizers, which are (though not if they are taken for less than six weeks). Tranquilizers may be prescribed if you feel so anxious that you cannot sleep and are becoming exhausted. Exhaustion makes everything, including any depression, worse.

Talking

Talking about your own feelings and having someone listen (really listen) to you with respect and sympathy can be healing and sanity-saving, especially if everyone has been focused on your baby's health most of the time. What you feel is immensely important and valid, and not just because you are the central person in your baby's life. You have a life too.

It helps greatly if, instead of bottling up your feelings, you can find someone you can talk to.

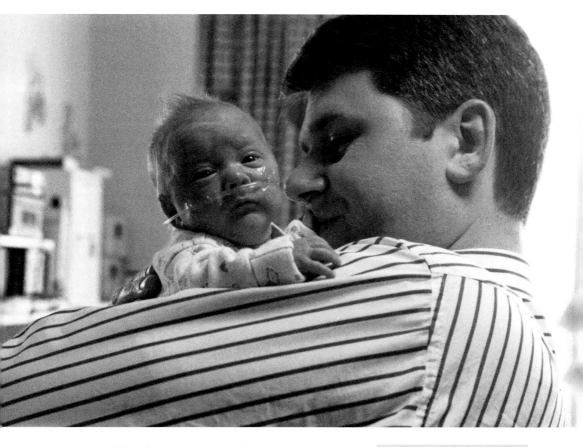

Naming your emotions

Having a baby can produce a wild range of powerful emotions in a parent, especially a new mother: you may feel wonderful, elated, happy, as if you rule the world, relieved, proud…or very vulnerable, fed up, depressed, shocked, and as if you can't cope with any of it. These feelings are all totally normal, and they do stabilize within a few days. But having a baby prematurely can make you feel even more emotional, and for a good deal longer. All your powerful instincts to cuddle, feed and care for your baby in the privacy, love and support of your own home may have no outlet. Your baby is so unwell you may not be able to hold her, and you are in an NICU where privacy seems non-existent. On top of all that you are likely very worried about your child's health and maybe even her survival.

Father and baby enjoying a cuddle

Keeping a journal is a positive and helpful way to channel your emotions and relieve stress. You will also be creating a special memento for you and your child.

Tips for eating

★ Always eat breakfast: research shows that this helps reduce stress and depression.

★ Treat food like fuel. Live off quick and easy-to-prepare foods that do the job fast and keep you going (such as instant oatmeal or granola, bananas, baked beans on toast, pasta and sauce).

★ Buy healthier take-out food that has plenty of carbo-hydrates, such as baked potatoes with fillings, and some salad with a carton of milk.

★ Buy high-energy snack foods and frozen meals in bulk so you never run out.

★ Keep some foods (such as fruit, crackers, quick noodle soups) in the NICU unit cupboard.

★ Eat at least one square meal a day in the hospital cafeteria. Try to pick an off-peak time, like before the noon rush starts, or after it's finished. Many hospitals have meal vouchers for parents staying all day.

★ Try to drink at least eight glasses (or more) a day of plain water, milk or diluted fruit juices. If you are not getting enough to drink, this can sap your energy further (and it is especially important to drink lots of water if you're breastfeeding). Tea and coffee make you urinate more, so you lose more vital water.

Many parents have said that recognizing and putting a name to or describing how they feel can help greatly. They also say they can remember feeling several different, powerful and sometimes conflicting emotions, ranging from blinding love, elation, obsession and hope to despair, anger, guilt and grief. They were in awe of their child, filled with respect and pity for her as she fought for life, fiercely possessive of her, and grateful to the NICU staff, but also powerless, isolated and shocked, blank and detached, bitter ("why us?") and resentful of the staff— sometimes a mixture of these just in one short visit to their baby, and some at seemingly inappropriate times.

Eating for energy

Many new mothers of a healthy term baby find they are so busy and tired at first that they seem to be living off breakfast cereal. And they don't have to spend hours each day at the NICU, as well as possibly having to juggle care of older children and a home, as you may be doing. But it is important to try to eat as regularly and healthily as possible, otherwise you will not have enough energy to be very much help to your baby, let alone for any other responsibilities you may have. The suggestions on the left all come from parents who have had premature babies.

Catnapping and rest

Just 15–20 minutes of complete rest or a catnap taken between 2 p.m. and 5 p.m. has a considerable "battery-recharging" effect. Try to find a place that's quiet and preferably off the unit for a quick but restoring mid-afternoon nap. Perhaps there is a parents' bedroom attached to the unit, or you may find that the parents' sitting room or quiet room is free at various times. Some parents kept a pillow and blanket in their car and went to lie down on the back seat for a quiet half-hour each day.

Getting help

Getting enough of the right sort of help can be quite difficult for a mother of a premature baby. One problem can be that, going home from hospital without a baby in your arms, family and friends don't treat you like a new mother who has only just given birth (and often in quite traumatic circumstances). In some cases, mothers have found that soon after they themselves came out of hospital their husbands were expecting dinner on the table, the housework done and any older children to be taken to and from school as usual.

However, many fathers want to do what they can for their partners, and may just need to be asked to do specific things—for example, your partner could be the one who makes the evening meal. This may be especially good if he does not like to spend much time at the unit itself at the moment, fearing there is nothing much he can do there for his baby (this is not true—see the previous chapter, *What can we do?*), but there is a lot he can do for you.

If you possibly can, try not to be too shy or independent to ask family or friends for a hand—nor too proud or embarrassed to accept it when it is offered. People often feel really good about being needed, and this is one time when you are entitled to all the back-up in the world. You can always return them some favors when things are easier.

If people do offer help, they may not know what would be the most use to you. Try to give them a few suggestions, such as food shopping, a dish (such as a stew, casserole or pie) dropped in so you don't have to make a meal when you go home, picking up older children from school and giving them snacks for a week, an hour of basic housework on a regular basis, or a ride to or from the NICU each day.

Surviving in the NICU

Just being in the NICU for so much time can be a stressful experience for parents. It's too hot, the lights are harsh, there is constant noise from alarms, phones, buzzers, and the commotion of frequent emergencies, day and night; and there is little or no privacy.

If you feel the staff are watching you, they probably are, but this is generally because they are trying to look out for unspoken signs from parents that they might need something—perhaps practical help, encouragement, or someone to talk to.

"I think I was more worried about Ashleigh. I didn't feel I could do much to help our baby at the moment. Yet Ashleigh I could help in important, practical ways. So I tried to support her by taking away the mundane tasks that she would usually have to worry about. I used to rush home from work, see her and our baby at the NICU for 45 minutes, rush home, look after Harry, our two-year-old, tidy the house, cook the evening meal…"

Mike, father of Scarlett,
born at 32 weeks

"Most of my friends had never even had a baby. They didn't know what to say to me so they didn't visit, and when they did, they'd say: 'What are all those wires then?' or 'Aren't you worried?' But two were great with the practicals. One gave me a lift each morning to the unit as I had no car, and my best friend did my laundry – just used to pick up the dirty stuff in the evenings, bring it back the next day clean and never even mention it."

Maria, mother of Gavin,
born at 34 weeks

"One thing we learned was: don't go looking into the incubators at other parents' babies! Respect their privacy. You may just mean to be kind in saying 'hello' to a baby who looks lonely. But it's not taken well if that baby is really ill. Or even if they are not that unwell but their parents are very protective or worried about them."

Trefor, father of triplets Tom, Ben and Megan, born at 29 weeks

"It's like being in a fish tank. The glass around you, the humming of machines, the heat and the closed-in, hot-house feeling, and I felt like everyone knew my business."

Maureen, mother of Nicholas, born at 34 weeks

"I have gone back to work three days a week as a nanny and I really feel like it's doing me good. The neonatal unit was my whole life for months. I have no partner to help take some of the pressure off. It's been so intense that I feel I really need another environment for a bit."

Louise, mother of Gabrielle, born at 24 weeks

Other parents may be watching you, too, perhaps out of sympathy because you are all in a similar difficult situation. They may just want to talk. They may be looking at you because they are very tired and feeling blank, so are staring vaguely at anything happening around them just as your eyes might stray to the TV. If your baby is ill, they may feel great sympathy but may also not know quite what to say to you.

Yet it is other parents who can be some of your greatest comforters and supporters at the NICU. They know at least part of what you feel because they feel it themselves, and are often going through very similar troubles with their own babies.

Privacy

It can be difficult to be with your baby in any kind of privacy, but it is well worth trying. Ask if there is anywhere where you and your baby could go quietly to just be together. If your partner is there, he might really like to have some peace and quiet with the baby or both of you. It can be the only time you feel you all belong together as a family.

If your baby is not well enough to come out of her incubator, ask if some screens could be placed around you both, while you sit by her.

Taking regular time out

You may find that you are spending almost all your time at the hospital. You may feel fine about this; or you may find that it is exhausting you, but you feel you ought to be there. If you can possibly manage it, taking time away regularly can make all the difference between coping and not coping. However, it's important that when you take time out from the NICU, however briefly, that you try to make it a real break. Some parents found, if they went home for a while, that unless they tried to do something specific such as watch a film on TV, they ended up sitting by the phone, worrying, instead of sitting by their baby's incubator, worrying.

Try to leave the NICU at regular intervals, even if it's just for half an hour to have a drink or a snack on your own in the hospital cafeteria. If you feel up to it, go for a short walk. It is also a good idea to find places other than the NICU where you can go regularly. If these places are in the fresh air where there is a chance of a little sun, so much the better: if you get out in daylight every day it helps your body make vitamin D (vital for healthy bones), estrogen (to help stabilize your hormone levels) and the feel-good chemical, serotonin. Or perhaps you can find an empty room or other private space—or even go and sit in your car for a while. Larger hospitals also have chapels, libraries or gardens where you can spend some time.

Asking for changes

Because you are likely to be spending more time with your baby than anyone else, you may be noticing many things about her that the staff, who change every shift, might not. Good neonatal staff understand and respect this.

If you feel that your baby needs a change in the way that the staff are caring for her, you will probably want to say so. Parents often find it difficult to bring up anything that could be interpreted as a criticism. But remember that she is your baby, and as her parents you do have every right to ask for changes that might make things better or more comfortable for her.

You and the neonatal staff are on the same side. You want the same thing for your baby—for her to get well—and you can make a great team. Yet in the end your baby does not belong to the NICU, she belongs to you, and it is your right to worry about your own child, to ask for things that might help her, to bring to the notice of the staff anything that you feel is the matter. Not only do you have powerful instincts as a parent, but you are not your average parent—one with a healthy term baby who has never yet had a day's serious illness. You are the watchful parent of a vulnerable premature baby.

If your early warning system is ringing but you sense that the staff might not really be listening to you when you tell them about it, you might want to look at the option of trying out a slightly different approach. Sometimes just the way a question or request is put seems to make a real difference to whether people take notice of what you say and try to help—or whether they don't.

"NICU parents are not ordinary parents. Some have been to hell and back. Some have spent days, weeks, even months sitting by an incubator, watching over their babies. Premature babies' parents understand the medical terminology, they know the complex equipment, the symptoms of many different types of disorders a premature baby can suffer from, and they know all about the treatments. Some have looked after a 2lb (0.9 kg) baby on a ventilator, others watched their children have repeated blood transfusions or even operations. Why shouldn't they worry? They have a right to. A premature baby's parent's own instinctive early warning system can save their baby's life."

Lisa Hollis, Hospital Community Neonatal Sister at Kingston Hospital, Surrey, England

Being tactful

Negotiating and being diplomatic take energy. When you are tired, worried, or not yet well yourself, energy is something you may be feeling very short of, and having to be a bit tactful might seem like the last straw, but it is worth it for your baby's sake.

137

"I thought if I said something about every single thing I wanted to mention, they (the staff) would think I was a real pain. I didn't want the nurses not liking me much to affect the way they looked after Sam. I wanted them to like me so that they'd be specially nice with him... so sometimes I used to not say things I wanted to say, like 'why has he been sitting in that dirty diaper for so long?'"

Karen, Sam's mother

"People may think you are a 'fussy' parent. Well, tough. You go ahead, you have every right. I tell mothers to be like a lioness protecting her cubs."

Anthony Kaiser, Consultant Neonatologist at St Thomas' Hospital, London, England

Jacky spends some quiet time getting to know Marina, born with her twin, Alex, at 24 weeks.

Perhaps try saying something like: "It would help me if you could…" rather than "I want you to…;" "What do you think about my baby having x, y or z?" rather than "My baby needs x, y, or z;" "I read this interesting idea, can I show you? What do you think about trying it?" rather than "Experts say/This book says you should…" Do try to comment on what was good first when you are asking for something to be changed: for example, "When my baby had a light blanket over her yesterday she seemed much more contented. Could we try that again today?" rather than "My baby doesn't like being without a covering. Where has her blanket gone?"

Try showing the nurses the things you have noticed that your baby likes. Ask if they have noticed this too. This can give you some common ground to discuss things from. Talk to other parents on the unit about what they did, how they got around certain problems. They may have found out which staff are more open to new suggestions, or found a good way through a situation similar to the one you are now trying to sort out. Ask if any of the senior nurses on the unit have regular meetings with the parents. This can be really helpful for pulling together all the information you need about how your baby is and getting certain questions answered and issues resolved, especially if you have been told different things by different people.

You need not accept being told: "No, we can't/don't do that" as permanent. Sometimes people hear something new and need to think it through, or consider what you said, before they can understand your point. Try giving it a day or so then ask again: perhaps something like "Do you still feel the same way about x? Perhaps you saw my baby doing y, as I mentioned the other day? Do you have a moment to talk about it again?"

"Difficult" parents
There are a few neonatal staff who do seem to feel that a "good" parent is someone who doesn't make any fuss: someone who doesn't ask too many questions all day, isn't around on the unit all the time, accepts what they are told and doesn't rock the boat. Don't worry if you don't conform to their no-trouble ideal of a good parent.

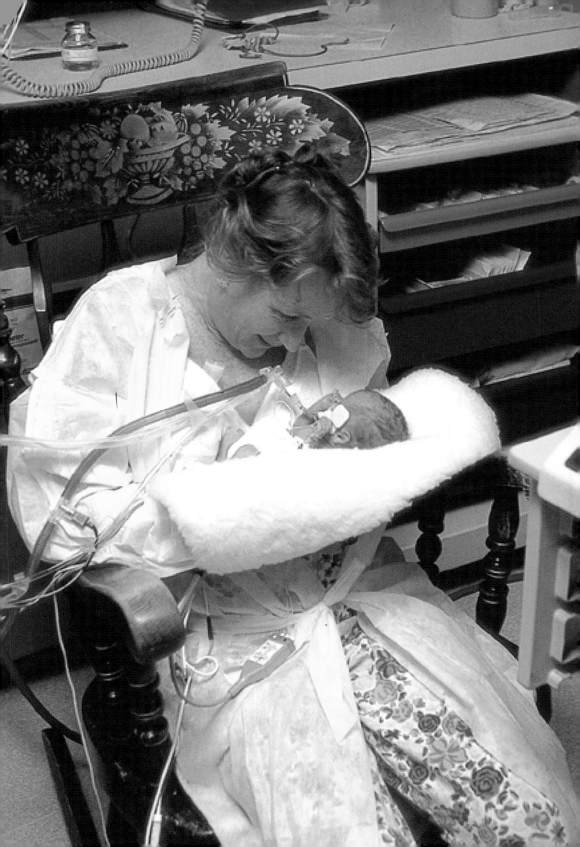

You need information

If you feel that the staff are becoming fed up with you because you ask too many questions, and this is bothering you, you could try saying something like: "I know that you are finding all my questions quite irritating. But I really need information. This is my way of coping. It helps me deal with things better. For me, knowing is much better than not knowing."

Keep a diary

Many parents do this, and say when they looked back over a couple of weeks they were usually really encouraged to see how far their baby had actually come, something that is easy to forget when you are living one day at a time.

Feeling at home

Most parents are made to feel welcome in their baby's NICU when they spend time there day after day, but a minority do say they notice a mixed reaction to their presence, especially if they are putting in long hours and appear to be "always there."

If this is the case for you and it worries you, try to have a quiet word with the nurse you feel the most comfortable with. If that does not get the results you need, try talking to a more senior member of staff on the unit about how you are feeling—perhaps the nurse practitioner, the psychologist, registrar, pediatrician or neonatologist—or one of the "support" staff such as the lactation consultant, social worker or minister.

Getting information

- Ask lots of questions—no question is too small. If you need to know something, then it matters. The chances are if you want to know about it, other parents will have too.
- If you can't catch the person you specially need to talk to, make an appointment. A nurse can do this for you. In particular, trying to catch the doctor to ask important questions while he or she is on rounds is not usually very effective. If you make an appointment for later, you will have some guaranteed uninterrupted time.
- Write things down (questions, points you want to mention). It can be easy to forget when you are tired.
- Ask for written summaries of complicated information. Doctors and senior nursing staff will be happy to do this for you. (Make sure you can read their writing.)
- If you are not sure what someone means, ask him or her to put it in ordinary words. Nurses and specialists get so used to using medical terminology that it is easy for them to forget that other people might find it confusing. However, parents often pick up the technical terms because they are so anxious to understand what's going on.
- Take someone with you if you think you could do with some moral support.
- Tape information-giving conversations so you don't have to take every detail in at the time. The NICU staff won't mind this.

- If you can't remember what a member of staff just said, it's OK to ask again—and again. No one minds. In fact, they'd be surprised if you didn't.
- Find as many books, information leaflets and so on as you can and read up on the subject. Most parents find this very helpful; others don't, and some couples find they prefer one of them to do the research while the other just focuses on coping with things as they come up.
- Don't settle for what sounds like vague, or incomplete information; this may only make you frustrated or more worried. Neonatal staff are very busy, and you might have to push a bit to get all the information you need.

YOUR BABY'S OLDER BROTHERS AND SISTERS

Introducing even a healthy, full-term new baby to her brothers or sisters can be traumatic, touching, funny, tentative or even something of a non-event as far as the sibling is concerned. Every child's response is unique, because no two children are alike. Nor are their feelings about having a new baby brother or sister. But if the new member of the family is a premature baby who may be fragile, ill or have special needs, this may intensify the older children's natural reactions, and might, for a while, cause repeated upheavals.

Brothers and sisters' reactions may depend upon how premature the new baby is, how well or unwell she is, how well their mother is and how much time she is spending at the hospital with the new baby every day. They may feel particularly displaced by a baby who, because she is premature, takes up so much of their parents' attention and who, as she is in hospital, may be physically removing their mother, or mother and father, from them and from their home for long periods. With older children especially, their feelings may be complicated and sharpened by worrying about the health of the new baby. Older brothers and sisters may not be any more accepting of a new premature baby than younger ones, and may miss a mother who is not able to be at home much almost as badly as a much younger child. They may also pick up more on any stress that having a premature baby is causing.

"He was about the size of a newborn kitten and his chest caved inward with every breath… This baby could not live, it was impossible. I know it sounds selfish, but I knew that I couldn't stay near him. I couldn't begin to love him because if I did I wouldn't be able to cope when he died… [However,] the more I saw him the more I forgot what I had thought on that first day. He didn't really do anything and his eyes were permanently closed, but I began to feel that he was a real person, and my brother… At the beginning they fed him through a tube, but when he got a bit better we could feed him with a bottle. I came up every evening at about six o'clock to give John his bottle."

Emily, who was 13 when her brother John was born at 24 weeks

When your children first meet the new baby

To help the meeting you might like to:

★ Tape a small present to the incubator as a gift from the new baby to her brother or sister. This tends to work best with toddlers but older children may appreciate the gesture too, even if they know it's from you.

★ Encourage loving contact by asking if they would like to stroke the baby's head, or put a hand on her back, or cup her head without touching it, or slide a finger into her hand for her to hold, or even, if she is well enough, hold her.

★ To lessen the impact of off-putting wires and tubes, explain simply what a couple of them are for, and let them trace the tube from the machine to the baby with a finger or with their eyes.

★ Ask if they would like to tell a story or sing a song to the baby, very softly. Explain that she may well already know and like their voices because she got used to hearing them when she was inside mommy's tummy.

Joseph is not very old himself, and a bit apprehensive, but his little brother is safe in his arms.

Helping your older children

However, at least you can often talk fairly straightforwardly to older children, explaining the situation and finding out about how they are feeling. Let them express their emotions and anxieties, and answer their questions honestly and don't downplay the seriousness of any illnesses your baby may have. At the same time, don't dwell on aspects that may make them fearful. Above all, constantly reassure them of your love and concern for them. Depending on how old and how capable they are, you may be able to involve them a little in their baby sibling's care, if they would like to and if she is well enough.

Even if your baby's siblings are very young, there are several strategies you can try to help them adjust. The advice given here is based on suggestions that parents of premature babies have said helped them with children under seven.

Meeting the new baby

When your children first visit, try to welcome them on your own. It will be easier for them if you don't have the new baby in your arms or very near you; then you can spend some loving time with them first, and all go together as a family to meet her. Some other suggestions from parents that might help this first meeting are given on the left.

Accepting the new baby

Help your children think of the baby as part of the family by calling her by her name, and referring to her as "our baby," "your baby" or "your baby sister." To help them feel the baby is a real part of their everyday lives, encourage them to take home something of the baby's—one of her bonnets, an old hospital name tag bracelet and, especially, a picture of her—which they can keep for themselves and show to their friends. You could ask them to make a picture of the baby or color a name sign that they could hang on the incubator, and they might like to draw a picture of themselves or choose a couple of photos of themselves to leave with the baby.

Ask your librarian for books written especially for young children about premature babies, which you could perhaps read together.

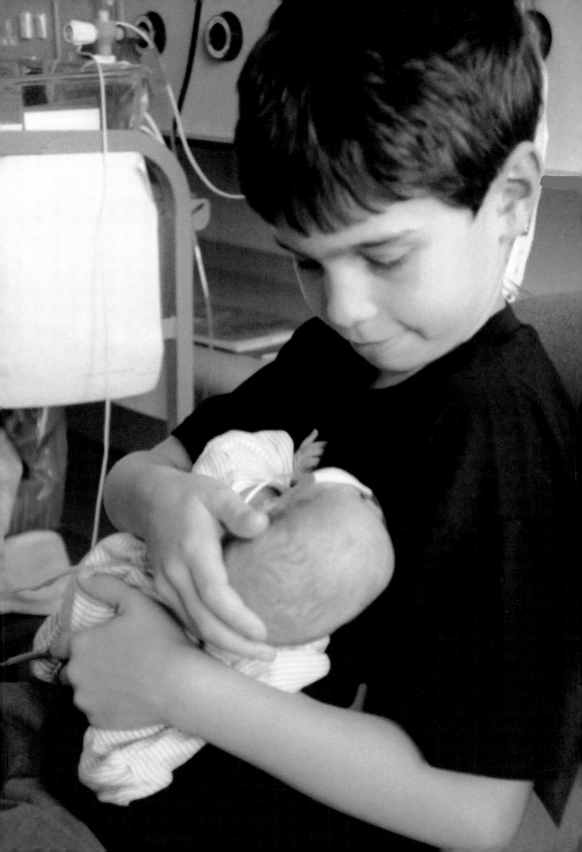

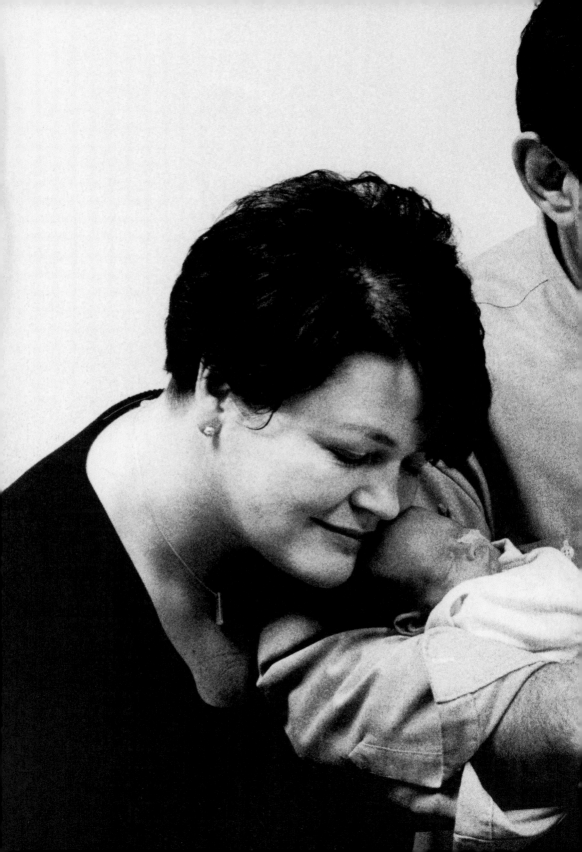

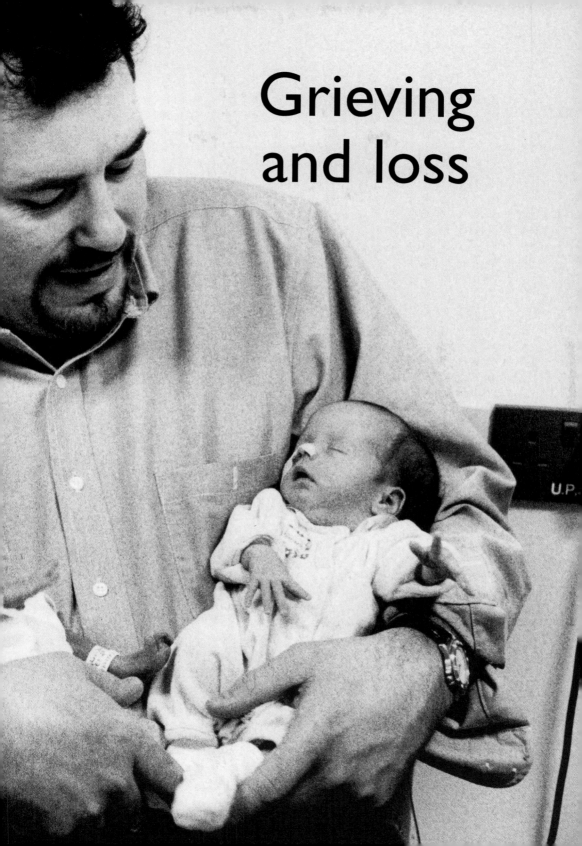

Grieving
and loss

"We had a little bedroom off the ward to ourselves and Tom was brought to us, still alive, on the ventilator. We were able to spend two or three hours with him, we dressed him ourselves, made him look nice."

Caroline and Trefor, parents of triplets Tom, Ben and Megan.

The photograph on the previous pages shows Caroline and Trefor with Ben and Megan, after Tom's death.

Grieving for a baby with a disability

Some parents, when they find that their baby has a disability, may grieve for the child that could have been. If a baby has a serious ongoing problem, the grief can be continuous, felt every time other children of the same age reach a developmental milestone that their child cannot manage: the stages at which they would usually be walking, talking, going to school, having a girlfriend, getting their first job, and so on. This grief is completely natural, too— many parents feel this way.

This chapter cannot possibly do more than touch the surface of some of the issues surrounding grief and a premature baby's death. But we are including it in the hope that it might possibly offer something of a starting point for parents who are thinking about seeking some support for the months ahead, because they know their baby is not going to live. It is also for mothers and fathers whose babies have died.

When a premature baby dies, nothing anyone says is going to take the pain and grief away. Yet often sensitive support from family, friends, doctors, nurses or counselors when and where you need it most, and for as long as you need it, can help you.

A premature baby who is very unwell may live for just a few hours, days, weeks or even several months. But it is not the length of the baby's life which forms the closeness: that love began in the uterus. Many parents say they felt bonded with their child long before he or she was born.

THE MANY FORMS OF GRIEF

Grief is a natural response when we lose something that is important to us. That is why parents of premature babies who survive sometimes experience it. They may be grieving for what they do not have—the full-term babies they had hoped for: the babies whom they longed to have in a crib next to the bed on the maternity unit like the other mothers did, the babies who did not need to be fed with the help of tubes, the ones who came home with their parents soon after they were born. The shock and distress of having a child prematurely can be enormous, and it is completely natural to mourn like this if your baby was born too soon.

The death of a baby

Grieving for a baby who has died is especially hard. The death of a baby is so shocking that the desolation and despair can be impossible to describe. It seems completely against the natural order of things for a child to die before his parents. People who have little experience of loss sometimes think that, since there is less to remember when a baby dies, there must be less to grieve for. Yet it can be, in part, the lack of memories that makes it so hard.

The more things you have, or can recall as memories of your child, the more you will have to remember and grieve for. What one of the nurses said to you one day as they helped you dress your baby; something your baby did; the doctors' words; photographs; your baby's clothing; his hospital wristband. All the small things that remind you of your child's short life and will always be important and special.

Most of us might think that grieving takes a few weeks and that the word simply means, as it is defined in dictionaries, "feeling deep sorrow." But it is more complicated than that, and goes on for longer than most people realize. Grieving is the very personal and necessary process that people go through after they have lost someone or something they love. Ultimately it is a healing process, too. Every person feels different things when they grieve. These feelings can and do change from day to day, and they may last a long time.

WHY GRIEF IS IMPORTANT

Time is said to be a great healer. But it is the process of grieving, as well as time passing, that helps to heal the pain of loss. Coming to terms with loss in this way does not mean forgetting the person who died. It involves remembering, and at the same time finding a permanent and special place for that person in your life, where it does not hurt you so much.

There is no "right" way to grieve. No one can possibly say to you: "Do this. You'll feel much better." Parents whose babies have died say that you have to find out what is right for you, then do it at your own pace. They also say that, with time, life does have meaning, purpose and joy once again, though you will never be quite the same person as you were before. They also say that it is natural still to feel and do things that you enjoy, to go out, enjoy friends' company and laugh again. But that this does not mean that you have forgotten about your baby, or that you are not still grieving inside.

Mourning that heals

William Worden, a Professor at Harvard Medical School who has worked a great deal with bereaved parents, says that there seem to be four main "tasks" of healthy mourning.

People do not necessarily experience these tasks in any particular order, or at any specific time. They are:

1 Accepting that what has happened is true.

2 Being able to feel and express your pain and emotions.

3 Gradually coming to terms with your altered life.

4 Being able to invest energy in life again.

As most people naturally experience these tasks of mourning, in their own time, and in their own way, there is no "correct" way to mourn the loss of a loved one. If you are experiencing feelings and thoughts that distress; and concern you, seek help from a trusted friend or professional counselor.

"I was as tired, as though I'd been working 20 weeks non-stop. I felt a terrible tense feeling inside me, almost as though I wanted to smash something up, simply because I'd lost my son."

Adrian, whose son Rikki was born prematurely, and lived for 81 days on a ventilator

What you can do for your dying baby

Depending on how fragile your baby is and whether he is on a ventilator or not, this could include:

★ Gentle touch or massage, if your baby might like it

★ Therapeutic touch

★ Talking softly to him

★ Containment care

★ Kangaroo care

★ Just holding him close to your breast

★ Everyday care: washing, diaper changing, dressing, comforting, and feeding even if it's by tube

★ Giving your baby breast milk, even if this is by tube

★ Staying by your baby so he can feel your presence

★ Leaving something small and soft that smells of you, such as a small scarf, in his incubator

★ "Thinking" love and calm into him

★ Arranging for your baby to be blessed or baptized

Feelings of grief

Just some of the powerful feelings parents say they remember having when their premature babies died include anger, and unbearable pain that seemed to go on and on—many people experience this as a physical pain too. They also mentioned isolation, loneliness, disbelief ("this can't be true") and denial, numbness, frustration, deep sadness, feeling a failure, depression, anxiety, physical tiredness and lack of energy, lack of appetite, loss of interest in sex, guilt, jealousy of pregnant women, of other couples with healthy babies. These feelings can be so powerful that many parents have said they became afraid that they might actually be going mad.

WHEN YOU KNOW THAT YOUR BABY IS DYING

Mothers and fathers who were able to help take care of their dying baby have said afterward that it helped them to feel they had done as much as they could for their child. Some parents find that caring for, and being physically close to, their dying baby feels natural, and that it is something they want to do. While for others, the fear and uncertainty create such anxiety that they pull away.

Many parents have said that they felt afraid of loving their baby when they knew he was not going to live. It is completely normal to want to distance yourself like this in the hope that it won't hurt so much when your child dies, and it can be very frightening not knowing what will actually happen. Yet it does not help to stay away. Bereaved parents have found that pulling away is, in the end, no protection from pain. In fact, the opposite is true. The less you are with your child, the more you may regret afterward. And wishing that you had been there more with your baby can be difficult to come to terms with later.

What can mothers and fathers do?

You can do many of the things you wanted to do when you were first thinking about having a baby to care for, and certainly most of the things described in *What can we do?* (see pages 84–127). In many ways, the more you can do, the more closely bonded you will feel, which is comforting both for you and for your baby. Talk to your baby's nurses about what you might like to do for him, about what would be possible, and whether they can help and support you in this.

You might like to save some of the clothes your baby has worn, so that his scent will remind you of him at home. And it is very helpful to keep a camera and to take as many pictures of your baby as you feel you might like— perhaps photos of him with you both, with any older brothers and sisters, or with the nurses. Some parents also take beautiful photographs of their baby's small hands or feet as mementos. (Polaroids give an instant result, but they tend to fade.)

If it is possible, try to involve your baby's grandparents and close family as well, encouraging them to come and visit and get to know your baby too at this very important time. The more people know your baby, the more they can begin to understand and help you. Visiting could help grandparents themselves too, as they may also be grieving doubly—both for you (because you are their child) and for their grandchild.

WHEN YOUR BABY HAS DIED

Many parents have said it helped greatly to be able to be with their baby when he died, perhaps holding their child in their arms. Sometimes parents help to remove gently any tubes and monitor wires afterward, then maybe wash and dress their child, or choose special clothes and other small belongings to go into the crib too. Other mothers and fathers remember they felt more comfortable when the nurse washed their baby after he had died, but wanted to come in and be with him afterward.

Gentle goodbyes

Many have said that having a photograph taken of their baby, perhaps with the whole family, including any brothers and sisters, together—perhaps with the nurse who knew their baby best too—was very comforting to look at later on. Nearly all mothers and fathers choose to spend some time with their babies afterward and need to

"I couldn't stop thinking about it. I went over and over the events of my baby's birth, illness and death in my mind in an endlessly repeating tape loop day after day, week after week. I couldn't stop, couldn't break out of it. I was obsessed. I thought: this is what it must feel like to go mad. I was so scared because I really thought I was going mad."

Anya, mother of Colm, born at 32 weeks

There is no "correct" way to mourn the loss of a loved one. If you are experiencing feelings and thoughts that distress and concern you, seek help from a trusted friend or professional counselor.

"I have always been a fairly gregarious person; and also quite a private person emotionally. I didn't show or talk about my feelings very often. I would never have imagined I would hold or hug a dead baby. But it seemed like exactly the right thing to do at the time. It helped us say goodbye to him. We loved him so much, even though he had only been with us a couple of weeks."

Trefor, father of Tom, Ben and Megan. Tom died in an NICU.

Children and funerals

Although in the past children were discouraged from attending funerals, it is increasingly being recognized that this kind of ceremony can help them in coming to terms with the death of a baby brother or sister. It is important to explain to them beforehand what to expect and what will happen. This could include letting them know that people will be sad, will say prayers and sing special songs for the baby—or anything else which you feel it would help your children to know about.

have space and time in a private room. This is also a special time when you, as a mother and father, can just be parents to your child.

The postmortem

Unless the doctors are quite sure about the cause of your baby's death, they will ask your permission to carry out a postmortem examination of his body. The pathologist who performs this may be able to find out if your baby was born with any particular physical problems. This could be vital information for any future pregnancies you may have.

A postmortem is done as carefully and delicately as if your baby were having an operation. You will be able to see him again afterward if you would like to. The procedure does not involve the hands or face, so most babies will not look very different from when their parents last saw them, except that by now their lips will probably be bluish, their skin mottled, and they will feel very cold to touch.

Some results of the postmortem may be available within a few days, others can take a few weeks. Parents are usually given an appointment in 4–6 weeks time, to meet their baby's specialist. She or he will be able to talk through any findings with you. It can be helpful to write down any questions you would like to ask as these can be hard to remember at the time. Some parents let the NICU know when this appointment is so they can also then come and see the staff again for a while.

The funeral

This is a way for you to say goodbye to your baby publicly. For some parents, it's important too because it can show how much their baby touched the lives of the people he came into contact with. A funeral can be arranged directly with the hospital chaplain, with your local minister or religious leader, or with a funeral director. Some parents choose to take their baby's body home before the funeral, which can also be arranged with the funeral director.

Feeling anxious

If your baby has lived for some time on the NICU before he died, you may find, as many parents have, that you feel isolated and anxious for a while afterward. Cocooned in that environment, you were protected as much as possible by the staff and, though extremely distressed, at least you felt supported by people who understood, and who knew both you and your baby. When you are back out in the world you can feel exposed and defenceless. It may help to know that this is completely normal, and an important part of any grieving process, but that it will pass and you will get your confidence back again.

"You may also find that friends and family may discourage you from doing something that you feel you would like to do. Try not to be put off. If it feels right to you, then it will probably help."

The Child Bereavement Trust

Other people

Some friends or family members can become your lifelines. Unfortunately, others, however kind they mean to be, are not always very sensitive or understanding and may say things that hurt you (usually because they are trying to make it better) or which miss the point.

"Would he have been badly disabled? Then it was probably just as well..." "But you've got two other lovely children," or "You can always try for another baby when you're feeling better." You may be very upset by such remarks, but try not to dwell on them. Other people may just not know what to say to you, and so avoid you for fear of upsetting you or sounding stupid.

Mothers and fathers grieve differently

The initial shock and sadness usually brings couples close to one another. But because mothers and fathers tend to grieve in different ways, the death of a child can put families and relationships under a great deal of strain as the months go by. It is very helpful if parents are able to share their feelings and support each other. When they can let each other in like this and say how they are feeling, this can help bring them close. If they cannot, there is a danger that it may tear them apart.

Fathers and mothers both feel the pain of losing their baby. But they tend to react differently and grieve for their child very differently. Bereavement groups have found that women usually feel better for sharing their pain and loss, for talking and crying, while men generally want to make things better, to restore and to mend. They are also usually very concerned about their partners.

Fathers often feel they need to keep away from pain, feelings and memories so they can help get things back to

Remembering

These are some ways in which parents whose babies have died have said it helped to keep a place for them in their and their family's lives:

★ Photographs: NICUs always have a camera and can take pictures for you or you can bring your own. Try to take as many photos as possible. Some parents find they don't want to have them at first, but feel ready to see them weeks, months, even years later.

★ Keeping a treasure box of mementos, or making something in memory of your baby: a painting, a book, a little corner of the garden or a window box, a pillow cover.

★ Thinking: perhaps there is a special quiet place you can go, a favorite park, or a church.

★ Talking to your partner about how you feel: make time to share any thoughts you have about your baby.

★ Sometimes it is easier to talk things through and be supported by someone who does not know you well, such as a counsel, a priest or, helpline (see page 203).

★ Marking anniversaries—a year after your baby's death, his birthday—in some way.

★ Planting flowers or trees in your baby's memory, perhaps with a special small ceremony.

★ A memorial service.

★ Making an entry in a Book of Remembrance at the hospital or crematorium.

normal as quickly as possible. So, many focus on supporting their wives from a practical point of view—doing the housework or shopping, taking any other children out a good deal, working to bring home the money, cuddling their partners when they cry. They do all they can to help practically, which is truly needed. But sharing the thoughts they have about their baby is needed too.

Men have often been brought up not to show their feelings. They are less likely to talk about their own emotions, and are afraid of upsetting or overburdening their partner further. They often fear that as she is so unhappy, saying anything about how they feel too may cause even more hurt. In fact, the very opposite is true.

Work is another major area of difference. Fathers are usually expected to be back at work within a very few days. Work colleagues may say they are very sorry to hear about what has happened—but then fairly quickly focus on work and the new shift/report/meeting/deadline coming up. Yet when fathers are back at home, they have to switch back into a completely different atmosphere, and often find the contrast difficult to handle day after day. For women, going back to work outside the home is usually an enormous milestone, when the only job they really wanted to have was to be at home caring for their baby.

Older brothers and sisters

It is completely natural for parents to want to protect their children from distress. But it is best to be honest with your older children if you possibly can. Parents who have been through this and professional counselors all advise that you should explain what has happened truthfully and simply. Children tend to imagine what you don't tell them to fill in the gaps, and what they make up is usually more worrying for them. It is better to use the word "died" rather than "lost" or "gone to sleep" or even just "gone," as psychologists have found that some younger children can fear that they might get "lost" forever too – didn't they get lost yesterday in the supermarket? – or that if they go to sleep at night they might never wake up again either.

What your older children can understand will vary greatly depending on their ages and how they are told.

From the age of two or three, young children can understand that their mother and father are sad because the new baby has died. But they will probably not be able to grasp the fact that death is permanent until they are older. It can help children of any age to be involved in saying goodbye to their baby brother or sister when you are all together as a family, so they feel involved and part of what has happened. Explain beforehand what to expect.

Some children find it natural to sit close to their parents and hold their dead brother or sister on their lap themselves, but offer them a choice and accept whatever they feel they would prefer to do. Many also choose to give the baby a small keepsake: ask them if there is anything they would particularly like to give. Some choose a toy they had been saving for when the baby came home.

Brothers and sisters of all ages will say their goodbyes in their own way. Perhaps by stroking the baby's head, kissing his cheek, patting his shoulder or laying a hand on the baby's tummy. They may welcome being asked if they want to help choose the baby's clothes, and make the incubator look nice. Some have helped a nurse take a footprint keepsake, or cut a tiny piece of hair. If one of the nurses is taking a photograph of your baby, older children often like to be there in at least one shot as part of the family.

It's fine to let your children see your tears too. They learn how to express their feelings by watching you. Be a little wary, however, of distressing them too much with your own painful emotions, as they may not know how to react. Children also need reassurance that you still love them very much, that you will still take care of them—and that you will not be this sad forever.

Your baby stays with you

Many parents find that after their baby has died, they have an ongoing and very personal relationship with him. Some say they often talk to their child in their heads, or like to go to a particular quiet spot to remember. Mothers and fathers often say that they see their child who died as part of their family, even if he was with them for just a short time. This is normal and natural: it is part of finding a way to hold on, even though you also let go.

Telling your children

It is best to be honest, and explain to children that:

* When people die, their bodies don't work any more.

* A dead person may look as if he is asleep but he is not, because when you are asleep your body works very well.

* When you die, it is forever.

* Because our baby has died, he will not be coming home with us. This has made mommy and daddy very sad.

"We are still grieving for Ruqiya. I don't think grieving ever stops for parents. She's a daughter of mine. I've got three daughters. Ruqiya is the eldest and she will always be remembered as the eldest."

Mohammed Aktar

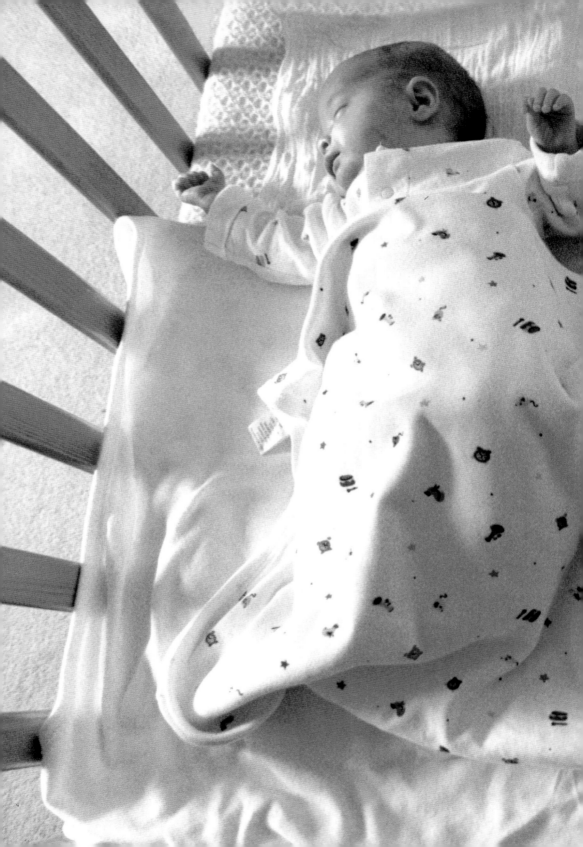

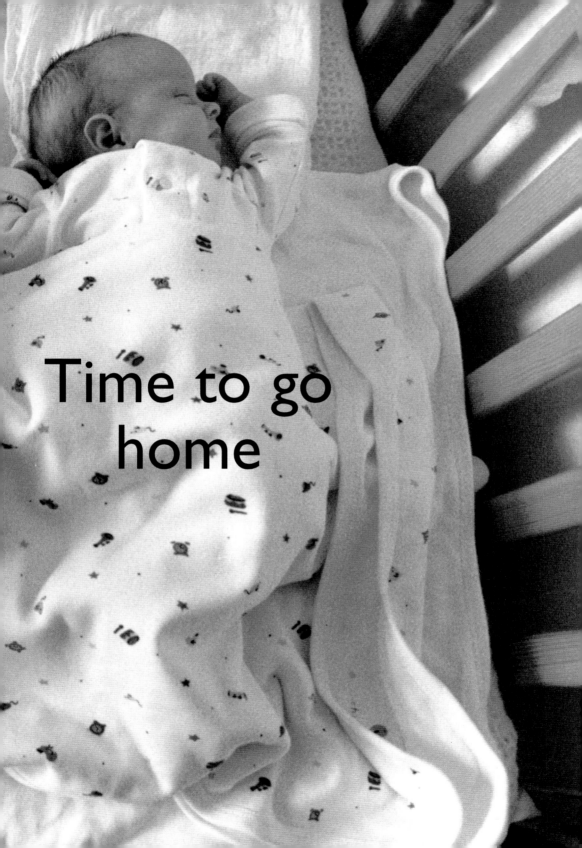

Time to go home

Beside feeling joy, celebration and relief to be home with their baby at last, many parents also say they can remember feeling a bit overwhelmed at first by the sheer logistics of looking after their premature baby when they first got home. Especially if they had other children to care for too and a home to run.

For many, getting into a routine, as baby- and childcare books recommend, was pretty much impossible, and they found the easiest thing to do was to take each day as it came, abandoning housework and cooking until they had the strength and energy. Yet many parents remember that after a chaotic few weeks, some sort of system did develop that suited them, even though it may not have been the organized routine of the hospital or the baby manuals. All new parents feel like this, but premature babies can be hard to look after, and their parents often have much more to cope with. Remember that there are many professionals—pediatrician, community services and the NICU—as well as helplines you can turn to for support and advice (see pages 163, 203). They are there to help you: don't be afraid to ask.

Looking good

Many parents mention how well their baby began to look in a remarkably short time. "She stopped looking like a pale, tired little hospital baby," as one father put it happily. And health workers who meet with mothers and their premature babies once they have returned home confirm that after about a week the babies' physical appearances tend to change dramatically. One said that "their eyes seem to sparkle, their body tone seems less floppy, they seem generally more robust, probably because they have been handled and held more. And, possibly thanks to their first bits of fresh air, their skin seems to glow."

HOW YOUR BABY MIGHT BEHAVE AT HOME

If your baby was born prematurely, she may at first mature at a different pace from term babies. She may also be a good deal more sensitive than a term baby for her first few weeks or months. The more prematurely she was born, the more you may notice this.

Corrected age

A baby who arrives early has two crucial dates that staff and parents use for measuring her progress. One is the day she was born, the other is her official due date, when she would have been in your uterus for around 40 weeks.

The time that has elapsed from the first date is her actual age: the time from the second date is her corrected age. When you are looking at what your baby is able to do (her developmental progress) you need to think about both these dates. Especially in the first year, the gap between them can make a great deal of difference to how quickly she matures, what she can cope with, and when.

After the first year, the gap usually becomes increasingly less obvious, as most premature children tend to catch up in their second or third years. However, what a premature baby is or is not able to manage to do or cope with also depends heavily on how well she is now, how well or unwell she has been since she was born and the way she was looked after in hospital. And all babies, including term babies, have their own personal "when I can do what" timetables, and these can vary a good deal.

Take, for example, two premature babies born at the same gestational age, having spent just 30 weeks in their mothers' uteruses instead of the usual 40. If one of them has had a difficult time (perhaps she had repeated infections, needed an operation and was on a ventilator for several weeks), she will probably not at first develop and mature as quickly or cope with as much as the other baby who only needed tube-feeding for two weeks and had just one minor infection. The baby who was more unwell will catch up, but it may take her longer.

Immaturity and sensitivity

For some months, premature babies may not able to cope with as much stimulation from, and interaction with, their world as term babies can.

Also, a term baby's behavior generally follows a fairly logical progression: For example, a term baby typically

---

**Actual age
– Number of weeks
   premature**

= Corrected age

You can work out your baby's corrected age from her original due date or by taking away the number of weeks or months premature she was from her actual age. So, if your baby is now five months old but was born two months prematurely, her corrected age is three months. Her level of maturity will probably—roughly—equal that of a three-month-old term baby. So she will not be able to do, or cope with, the sort of things that a five-month-old baby usually does.

"Half the time, I never knew what was coming next. He'd start screaming out of the blue, fall asleep abruptly when I was trying to sing to him, cry his head off for no reason in the middle of a nice feed. Thanks to our community neonatal nurse, I eventually accepted that I wasn't doing anything wrong, that was just the way Richard was at that time. It took a good six months for him to settle down."

Sue, mother of Richard, born at 29 weeks

Differences between premature and term babies

Every baby is an individual, but in comparison with normal term babies, premature babies just home from hospital seem to:

★ At first, prefer less noise, less excitement, less playing with, less eye contact, and need a much calmer quieter life.

★ Find it harder to calm and comfort themselves.

★ Change their behavior and mood very suddenly.

★ Be more time-consuming to look after.

★ Be noisy sleepers.

All these characteristics are normal for babies born early. The earlier they were born, the more noticeable these things are.

This is because their nervous systems did not get the chance to finish developing and fine-tuning in the uterus, and this process will now take a bit longer than if they were still protected inside their mothers with nothing else to do but mature.

Babies and sleep

Although babies are "supposed" to be sleeping through the night by six months, according to the ongoing *Children of the 90s* survey being conducted in the United Kingdom, in reality, only 16 percent of *term* babies are doing so, let alone babies who were born early.

will go from quiet sleep where she moves very little to alert sleep where she is more active and coming close to waking up, then be awake but dozy, then fully awake and alert, then begin to fuss and cry a little and progress to full-blown crying until someone does what she needs (maybe change her wet diaper, pick her up and cuddle her, feed her). A premature baby, however, tends not to follow a consistent pattern and so it can be difficult for parents to care for her because their baby's behavior seems so unpredictable. She may wake suddenly screaming from a deep sleep. She may be feeding quite calmly one minute, then drop into a deep sleep with no warning drowsy period in between. Or go from feeding happily to a desperate crying fit for no obvious reason. This can make it harder to cope with or to know what to do next, but it is normal behavior for babies born prematurely, until their systems settle down.

SLEEPING

Difficulties with sleep are very common with all new babies—and with older ones for that matter—but premature babies often have particular problems, and although they may spend more time asleep than term babies, they tend to sleep for shorter periods.

Reasons for sleep problems

Premature babies have been used to the bustle, bright lights and constant noise of the NICU. At night NICUs are still very busy, and so far your baby has been trying to sleep in the atmosphere of that unit. She may be unsettled by the quiet and darkness of your home at night.

Another cause of sleep problems is that a premature baby's small stomach may only be able to take small amounts of milk at first. This does not satisfy her for long and she may wake every couple of hours needing more. By the time you have fed and re-settled her, and got yourself back to sleep, it may be only another hour or so before she wakes again.

All babies go through natural growth spurts and periods when their nervous systems mature especially fast, and the same is true for premature babies, though their timetables for doing this may be rather different. This can temporarily make a baby less settled and disturb her sleep patterns for a while.

Helping your baby to sleep

As a premature baby's stomach grows bigger and can hold more milk, and her neurological system becomes more mature, she will sleep increasingly well at night. There is also quite a bit you can do to encourage this.

For instance, if your baby is unhappy with silence and darkness, leave a bedside light on near her crib to begin with, to wean her gently from wanting to go to sleep with the light full on. Later you can move the light further away, and then replace it with a dim night light. Have the radio on quietly at night, turning it down a little more each day over a period of weeks. You are trying to show your baby

A double feeding, at home

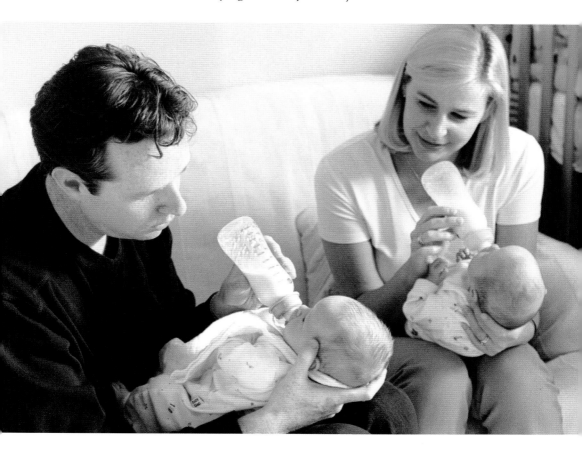

"When I took Rohan home he would scream and cry if he was in the dark, so I left a gentle night light on in the corner of the room. He didn't like it being so quiet either so for weeks we had the radio on all the time, gradually turning the volume down until there was first quiet white noise, then silence."

Meera, mother of Rohan, born at 28 weeks

Soothing tactics

You could try:

★ Wrapping or swaddling your baby snugly and holding her comfortingly close to you as you stay still and quiet

★ "Wearing" your baby in a sling around the house so she stays close to you all the time, or kangaroo care (see pages 104–107).

★ Resting somewhere quiet in dim light with your baby lying on your chest with her ear near the comforting, calm beat of your heart

★ Containment care (see page 100).

that night and day are very different (term babies need to learn this too) so during the day you might like to keep the lights on or the curtains open and a bit of background noise going and interact with your baby as much as she can cope with. At night, try to feed her in a quiet, calm and cozy atmosphere and keep everything low key. If your baby needs changing, try to do this as she lies quietly in her crib rather than taking her out of it or into another room. Keep lights dim and sounds down if you can, and try to keep any interaction with your baby to a gentle minimum.

It can also help to get into some sort of routine when you are able to. It does not have to be strict, just one where certain things—a feeding, a car ride to take older children to school, a bath, a stroller walk, another feeding—happen more or less at the same time, to give each 24 hours a bit of (flexible) structure. If you can possibly manage to do this, after a while, it will help teach your baby the difference between night and day too. Routines can have a very calming effect on the entire family. But it is far easier to establish a routine with some babies (premature or full term) than others.

If your baby often wakes with hunger, try offering a little more milk in the last night feeding. If your baby is being breastfed but is used to occasional bottles of formula as well as your breast milk, giving a formula feeding last thing at night may help her sleep a little longer, as it takes longer to digest than breast milk.

Minimizing your sleep disturbance

If your baby sleeps right next to your bed, flush up against the side, it is easier just to lean over, scoop her gently into bed with you to feed her, then put her back into her own bed with minimal disturbance to either of you. If you do not have to get up out of bed to go to her you can do this when only half-awake and get back to sleep more easily. This is easier if you are breastfeeding. Keep basic diaper-changing material by the bed too, so if necessary you can change a wet diaper as your baby lies snugly next to you (a dirty diaper will probably need a trip to the bathroom).

CRYING

Babies in general cry more than anyone thinks. At six weeks, crying for up to four hours a day is within normal limits for term babies. If you add up all the five- and 15-minute chunks in which crying tends to happen, even the average time is a couple of hours, which is actually quite a lot. So it is not surprising that babies who were born early, and were that much less mature to begin with, may cry for two to four hours every day for longer than the "usual" six weeks after birth. Just how much longer can depend on how early your baby was born, and how much catching up her nervous system and general development still have to do, and also on how ill she has been, how well she is now and how peaceful her environment is at home.

Crying is normal—it may even be a healthy sign. Research suggests that all babies' nervous systems go through several important stages of development in the first year of life, and it is thought that each time a baby's system goes through these developmental jumps forward, she may be more unsettled, cry more and wake up more often at night.

Calming a crying baby

There are many ways to try and calm a crying baby who was born at full term. You probably know them already. In fact, if you have other children, you are probably an expert and will have successfully used many stop-crying tactics in the past: back-patting, rocking, singing, dancing holding the baby, distraction with toys or making surprise faces.

Yet these techniques do not seem to work on a crying premature baby, even when she is well and strong enough to be home: the usual baby-soothing combination of movement, sound and sights can be too much and she will probably cry even more. Some early-born babies are overwhelmed and upset by cheery faces talking up close to theirs, being bounced up and down, or being sung to, rocked and patted all at the same time.

This may be because they are still finding it difficult to handle more than one thing happening to them at once—especially if they are already upset. Perhaps you have already noticed that, say, sitting still and holding your baby

Is your baby in pain?

Sleep problems and excessive crying can also be caused by medical problems. Is your baby:

⋆ Swiping at, or even pulling at her ear or the side of her head? She may have an ear infection.

⋆ Not wanting to lie down flat? It could be GER (see page 166) if it's after a feeding, or stomach pain, or an ear infection.

⋆ Sleeping badly, crying, and very jumpy? She may have a headache.

A headache may be something to do with her actual birth. If your baby was born vaginally, this may have compressed the soft bones of her skull a little and this compression can sometimes affect the pressure of the cerebrospinal fluid that circulates around her spinal cord and brain. Compression may also occur if she has a degree of head flattening (see page 97).

Noisy sleepers

A sleeping premature baby can make a remarkable amount of noise for someone so small—something you are unlikely to find out until you go home, unless you have roomed-in with your baby in hospital.

You do eventually get used to it though and usually sleep through it, only waking if there is a different note to the noises, for example a hungry whimper.

"When we first got home I had Megan in what I thought was a snug four layers of clothing, tucked up under blankets in a basket. She promptly developed a temperature so I called up the NICU in a panic. 'Just take off a few layers, and take her temperature again in half an hour' said the nurse calmly. I did. Sure enough, it went right back down again."

Caroline, mother of premature Megan and Ben

Taking your baby's temperature

It is a good idea to learn how to do this while still on the NICU. The most accurate way is using a digital thermometer: place it underneath the baby's armpit, and leave it in place for three minutes. The average normal temperature is 97.9–98.8°F (36.6–37.1°C).

Checking by touch

It is also useful to be able to judge your baby's temperature by touch. Every day for a week, take her temperature, then lay your hand on the back of her neck or on her tummy (hands and feet are not accurate guides). You will soon learn to recognize what she feels like when her temperature is a bit cool, say 96.8°F (36°C), or slightly raised, perhaps 100.4°F (38°C).

close to you with the radio turned right down can help settle her. Yet walking back and forth as you firmly pat her back and sing her a nursery rhyme (a time-honored way of soothing crying term babies) only makes her worse.

Crying babies with staying power can and do wear the most robust and calm parent to a frazzle. If you are worried about your baby's crying or are finding it difficult to cope with, try to get some practical and moral support. Try talking to other mothers of premature babies who know what this is like, to your midwife, community neonatal clinic (if you have one) or pediatrician—or, if you have very recently come home, the hospital's neonatal unit, where people will remember you and your baby.

Try to be as flexible as you can—what works one day may not work the next. And be confident that it is not going to spoil your baby if you pick her up when she cries—no matter what anyone else says about not "giving in" to her. Most importantly, try not to feel guilty or blame yourself in any way: having a baby who cries a lot does not mean you are a bad parent. In fact, you are a really exceptional and very special parent who is having to cope with a situation that most ordinary mothers or fathers never need to handle. Most parents of premature babies have gone through more, work harder, know more, and have built up an incomparable fund of special skills, stamina, faith and patience. If you can, try to make a little regular time for yourself and ask for and accept help so you can have short breaks. Hold on to the fact that your baby will settle eventually, and that in the long term it does get easier as your baby matures.

KEEPING WARM

By the time your baby comes home, she will usually be reasonably good at controlling her own body temperature. As she becomes chubbier, it is easier for her to stay warm.

Many parents worry about their babies getting too cold, as they may still seem so small and fragile, and they often have chilly hands and feet. It can be tempting to dress a small premature baby recently back from the NICU in a thick sleeper, then pile the blankets or baby duvet on top of that. However, while you do not want your baby to get cold, it is equally important to make sure she does not get too hot, as this can increase the chance of crib death (see page 172).

Don't feel your house should be as warm as the NICU, where the babies were sick. Your baby is now well enough to be in your home. She is bigger, stronger and more mature than she was, and so better at controlling her own body heat. Generally, you should try to keep the room she is in at around 63–68°F (17 to 20°C). Position her crib away from any radiators or heaters.

It is best to dress her in light layers, so that if she feels too warm to you, you can remove one layer at a time, checking her temperature after a few minutes. Be guided by how warm or cool you are feeling. If you are comfortable in a short-sleeved top or a light dress, your baby will probably only need a cotton vest and sleeper with feet, a light cotton cardigan and perhaps a cotton (not nylon) bonnet.

Make up her bed, too, with several thin layers of bedding (cotton blankets and sheets) rather than a baby quilt. If you find you need a sweatshirt indoors, tuck a double layer of light cotton blanket around her.

Very small babies

If you are taking home a little premature baby who only weighs around 4 pounds (2000g), she may still need to be kept a bit warmer than bigger babies. Before you go home check with the neonatalogist or pediatrician as to how many layers you can safely wrap your baby up in, both in her crib and out of it.

ADJUSTING TO LIFE AT HOME

Your first few weeks or even months after bringing your baby home from the NICU can be a bit disorienting. Most parents of premature babies remember that, at first, even simple everyday things, such as having a friend over or going to the supermarket can seem too much to cope with.

Community support services

Depending on where you live, there will be a number of services available to help you adjust at home. Ask your doctor about:

★ home visit by a nurse within 48 hours of your baby's discharge

★ phone communication with community or hospital nurses

★ continued home visits by a community or hospital outreach nurse

★ postpartum clinics where you can "drop-in" for problem-solving, health assessments, referrals, support or advice

★ physician follow-up within 7 days of discharge for the baby and 6 weeks for the mother

★ community maps to help new parents locate support services

★ breastfeeding clinics or centers and home visits by lactation counselors

★ parenting support groups or classes

★ homemaking services including cleaning and prepared meals

★ social worker support services

A moment of relaxation for mother and baby

Dealing with visitors

Parents' tried and tested visitor tactics include:

⋆ Being honest if now is not a good time.

⋆ Sometimes ignoring the door bell.

⋆ Getting a cheap answering machine so you can choose whether or not to answer once you've heard who it is and why they are calling.

⋆ Asking your partner to let friends know you would like to see them (if you would) but that you are very tired, so please could they, as one mother put it: "Take me as you find me, make your own tea, bring your own biscuits, stay half an hour at most and please call first."

"When Scarlett was crying incessantly and Harry was playing up, getting out of the house with the stroller was the thing that saved our sanity."

Ashleigh, mother of Scarlett, born at 32 weeks

"It was all so much trouble the first few times, I nearly stayed at home."

Vishnu, mother of Shreyas, born at 33 weeks

Visitors

Everyone handles being newly back home with a new baby (or babies) differently. However, most new parents, whether their baby was born early or at term, say they would rather not have visitors constantly popping in, as their first priority is their baby, their family, and getting their own balance back.

If visitors offer help, try to accept if you possibly can. If you find that you are too tired and muddled to think when people ask what they can do for you, keep a "helping-out list" with, for example, shopping, cooking, laundry, picking up or taking other children to and from school, to remind you and show them what you need.

You may also find you would prefer to limit how much even the nicest visitors handle your baby. Polite discouragement tactics suggested by parents include wearing your baby in a sling close to you or securing her in a baby seat and seeing she stays there.

Out and about

It can feel like wonderful freedom and blessed normality to do something even as simple as go out with your baby in the stroller after so long in the NICU. But the sheer mental effort of getting out with your baby can also seem quite intimidating at first, especially if you are tired and have been very stressed. You may not be used to being outside much yourself, either, if you have spent weeks or months mostly at the NICU. You may worry that your baby will catch an infection and, not surprisingly, fear crowded places such as play groups and stores for this reason. Many mothers remember feeling overwhelmed by all the bits and pieces of equipment to take, and all the organization. Some fear the logistical difficulty of using public transport, while others worry about car safety.

You might like to wait a couple of days after coming home from hospital before you first go out. Parents often say they did this so that their babies could get used to their very different new environment before introducing them to anything else. Why not try starting small, with say, a 15–20 minute stroll to the park or around the block. Then

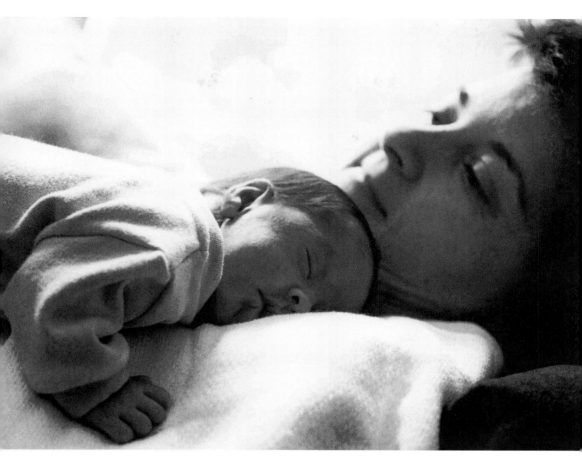

work up to more complicated outings, for example a trip to a mother- and-baby clinic, or a supermarket run.

It also helps to make a list of what you might need for trips, and have essentials permanently in the diaper bag and hoods and raincovers handy for your stroller. Leave at least half an hour after a feeding before traveling by car or bus, to reduce the chance of your baby being sick, especially if she has any digestion problems.

IF YOUR BABY IS ILL

You may well need to take your baby back into hospital because she has become ill at some time during her first year at home. In fact a premature baby is up to five times as likely to need re-admitting as a baby who was born at full term. Research suggests that between one-quarter and

"When Scarlett became ill I had to take her to our own doctor twice and to emergency twice (all in the same four days) before she was admitted. It turned out we were right—in fact, she had pneumonia. Premature babies' parents have to trust their own good instincts about their babies. Don't be put off if the doctors make you feel like a child being told off for making a fuss by a teacher."

Ashleigh, Scarlett's mother

165

Common signs of illness

Telephone your doctor, midwife or community nurse if you notice any of the following signs, or, if you are really worried, go straight to the Emergency Room.

1 Your baby just doesn't seem right to you—she may be behaving differently, be less active than usual, have a different note in her cry, be harder to wake up.

2 She has a temperature of over 100.4°F (38°C); or a temperature raised slightly but less than this plus other symptoms.

3 She is not eating.

4 She has fewer wet diapers.

5 She is vomiting most or all of her food.

6 She is crying more than usual, or is irritable.

7 She won't sleep, is fighting sleep, or is clearly tired but cannot seem to fall asleep.

8 She has diarrhea.

9 She has breathing problems: pulling her chest muscles right in, breathing noisily, breathing harder or faster than usual.

10 There is a change in her skin tone: she may be paler, mottled, bluish.

11 She is limp, listless.

12 She does not like you to touch or move her or shows discomfort when you do.

one-half of all premature babies need to go back into hospital for a spell during their first year, compared with around one in ten term babies. The most usual reasons are long-term health problems including BPD, heart and digestion problems, hernia repairs and infections.

If you think your baby may be ill, trust your own instincts. If you are really concerned, take your baby to the emergency department of the nearest major hospital. Staff there should always take a potentially sick premature baby seriously, but you may need to be persistent if you sense your baby is ill but this is not yet obvious to the hospital.

Good doctors and nurses know to listen to parents, and they respect mothers' and fathers' judgments of their own baby's well-being. But if you feel something is definitely wrong yet no one is taking it seriously you may just have to nag and pester. You know how your baby is if she is unwell, you have probably seen it before, so persist.

Avoiding infection

In their first year of life a premature baby is especially vulnerable to throat, lung and other breathing infections and also to ear infections. However, there are various ways in which you can reduce the risk. Make sure anyone who handles, picks up, touches or feeds your baby has newly clean hands every single time, whether they are a visitor, an older brother or sister or parents. If at all possible (though this is easier said than done), try not to take your premature baby into crowded enclosed spaces such as rush-hour buses and trains, supermarkets on a Saturday morning, packed mother-and-toddler groups, very busy play groups, school classrooms and parties, at least for the first months. If you take her to the pediatrician or clinic, try to get the first appointment of the day before the waiting room fills up.

GASTROESOPHAGEAL REFLUX (GER)

GER is similar to the heartburn that adults can develop. It is common in premature babies—the more premature they are, the more likely it is that they will have GER for a while.

If a premature baby has GER, the ring of muscle that separates the stomach from the esophagus (gullet) is too weak to remain closed, as it is supposed to. This means that partially digested milk and burning stomach acids can find their way up from the stomach where they belong, into your baby's throat. This is called regurgitation. When a baby regurgitates because she has GER, she may also gag, stop breathing for a moment, then start coughing and choking. This tends to happen (if it is going to) during or after a feeding or when your baby is lying down asleep, especially if she is on her back.

GER can be miserably uncomfortable and, in some severe cases, if it has not been spotted and treated, the baby's esophagus can develop painful ulcerated patches from the stomach acids. GER can also make it difficult for a baby to feed happily or to keep her milk in her stomach afterward. This then makes it harder for her to gain weight or grow well.

If it is not tackled, the regular discomfort of GER each time she feeds may also make it generally difficult for a baby to enjoy eating. It may even create a dislike or in extreme cases a fear of eating and swallowing food that may carry on well into toddlerhood and early childhood.

The good news about GER

GER tends to disappear as your baby spends more time upright—first sitting up alone, then toddling and walking. This is partly because her overall muscle-tone is improving, including that of the ring of muscle separating stomach from esophagus; and partly because, as she remains more upright, gravity helps to keep the food down instead of allowing it to come back up.

What parents can do to help

In general, if your baby has GER, it helps to keep her as upright as possible most of the time. Try walking around holding her against your shoulder, or sit with her lying up against your shoulder on her tummy. At night, you could try semi-reclining in bed with your baby stretched out comfortably on her front with her head on your shoulder and feet pointing down toward your waist.

Managing GER

★ Feed your baby with her sitting upright or at least semi-upright and make sure she stays upright for about half an hour after each feeding.

★ Feed slowly, taking several breaks and rests; or feed her less milk at a time, but more often.

★ Change your baby before, rather than during or after, her feeding and make sure her diaper is not too tight around her stomach.

★ Raise up the head end of your baby's crib or cradle so it's at about a 30-degree angle. A stroller whose sleeping position you can adjust to the same angle may be very useful here too.

★ Check your baby does not have problems digesting milk protein (lactose intolerance). Ask your doctor, pediatrician or midwife about this.

★ If your baby is bottle-fed, check to see whether the formula milk powder you are using is based on casein. Some health experts recommend this should not be used for premature babies even when they get older, as it can be hard to digest.

Signs of possible breathing trouble

If your baby is:

* Breathing faster than usual (approximately 60 or more breaths a minute)

* Having to work hard to breathe, pulling her chest in very noticeably (doctors call these retractions)

* Wheezing

Any of these may signal the early beginnings of a respiratory infection. See or speak to your doctor that day. If he is not helpful, or your baby becomes worse, call him again, or go to the emergency department of your local hospital.

These tips may help sniffly premature babies. Try:

* Damp-dusting all surfaces

* Washing any removable furniture covers

* Washing any furry household pets, especially cats (difficult to do, but many asthma specialists believe that cats, and to a lesser extent dogs, are asthma sensitizers)

* Keeping a runny nose clear by using a soft tissue

"When the NICU first suggested the idea of taking Mark home while he was still oxygen-dependent, I thought—I don't know, I'm not a nurse. I can't do this. But we did. And it was the best decision we ever made."

Catherine, mother of Mark, born at 32 weeks, who had chronic lung disease

If you can, try not to focus too much on your baby's weight gain at the moment. This can be a major worry for parents whose babies have GER. Yet if your baby is otherwise well, and being monitored by both you (who know her best) and good health professionals, you are doing all you need to at the moment. See if you can handle the GER by gently managing the way your baby feeds or sleeps, because that just may be all you need. But if you feel that some medical help is called for, see your pediatrician or baby clinic. They will probably prescribe a medicine to reduce the levels of acid in your baby's stomach and/or one to speed up the rate at which it empties itself of food (so there is less sitting there waiting to come back up again).

BREATHING PROBLEMS

In their first year at home, premature babies tend to have more respiratory (breathing) infections than term babies. If your baby has had BPD and was on a ventilator or had long-term breathing support she will be more vulnerable to this type of infection. Colds, s stuffed nose, coughs and sore throats can be thoroughly uncomfortable and may interfere with sleeping or feeding, but they are usually not serious. Occasionally, however, what appears to be a minor infection can develop into a more severe illness, such as bronchitis or pneumonia, so it is a good idea to keep a careful eye on your baby if she does get a cold. Breathing infections are among the most common reasons for readmitting former NICU babies to hospital during this first year.

The sniffles

At the milder end of the scale, premature babies are often very sniffly when they first come home. This could just be a reaction to ordinary house dust and should pass in time as your baby gets used to dust mites and stray pet hairs.

If your baby seems to be otherwise healthy and is feeding well you can ignore persistent sniffling for the moment and carry on as usual. But if she has had support from oxygen therapy at home (see below) and develops this type of condition, keep a close watch. If she develops a respiratory infection, even a cold, she may need oxygen therapy again for a while to help her recover.

COMING HOME WITH OXYGEN

Babies who need extra oxygen but are otherwise well, stable and have reached a reasonable weight may be allowed home if their parents can learn and feel confident about the care and equipment they will need.

A premature baby may need this extra help for just a few months but in some cases the time-scale is a few years. This may sound a bit daunting, yet most parents who have done this say they did not find many problems with using the equipment once they become used to it. The NICU staff will show you how to operate the oxygen machinery until you are confident with it, and arrange for it to be installed at your home.

Once you are all home, you can keep in close touch with your baby's pediatrician for support and to help with any difficulties you may experience. Your baby will assess your baby regularly, to see how she is doing and whether the amount of oxygen she is being given can be gradually reduced.

You would probably be using either oxygen cylinders, or a device called an oxygen compressor or concentrator, which separates the oxygen out of air and feeds it to your baby. As the concentrator runs on electricity, you would also have a portable back-up oxygen tank to use when you are out and about, or in case there is ever a power failure.

Some NICUs will allow parents and their premature baby to share a room attached to the unit for a night or two, before they all go home together, so that the parents can become used to being "in sole charge" while still having the reassurance of knowing the staff are there if they need them. If your baby is going home still needing oxygen, you might like to room in for a couple of nights or so to give yourself time to become comfortable with using the cylinders or compressor too.

The most common reason for a premature baby to graduate from the NICU to her home still needing oxygen

The benefits of home oxygen therapy

If a premature baby needs oxygen therapy, it can sometimes be a long time—up to as much as four years from the time she began—before she is weaned off extra oxygen completely. Giving her oxygen yourself means that, rather than spending that time in hospital, your baby is at home where you can be a family together. At home, premature babies thrive and grow better, are happier, eat better and are less likely to pick up infections than they would in hospital. And you won't have to be constantly torn between being at the hospital and home.

Oxygen therapy: cautions

* Oxygen is highly flammable. Keep your baby and all oxygen supplies well away from any flames, such as an open fire or a gas appliance with a pilot light.

* Absolutely no smoking in the room where the oxygen equipment is kept.

* Keep your baby away from smoky atmospheres.

* Make sure your home is fitted with smoke detectors—and that they work.

* Keep the door of the room open so it does not become stuffy.

Weight gain—how much is enough?

"Ideal" weight gain for a new baby is about 1oz (28g) a day, but a premature baby may not be putting on this much, especially if she has a condition affecting weight gain, such as BPD (see page 61) or GER (see page 166).

Talk to your pediatrician or neonatologist about the sort of weight gain they feel is enough for your own baby. Check how much weight she is putting on using a baby weight chart. (Ask your doctor for one.) You may also find one of these in her medical records or in her book record of health. If she is below the bottom percentile (that is, the band with the lightest weights) but running parallel to it rather than dropping away, that's usually enough.

Common tube problems

★ Irritation, soreness or a little bleeding around the nostril that the tube goes into. A little petroleum jelly can help protect against this. The tube can also easily be changed over to the other side while the sore nostril heals.

★ Occasionally the tube may cause irritation or soreness in the throat. If you do notice a little blood (perhaps when your baby brings up some milk) let her doctor know.

★ When the tube is put in or removed, it may make a baby gag, or vomit briefly.

support is that she was born before 32 weeks and has BPD—chronic lung damage (see page 61). The good news is that as your baby grows so does new lung tissue, and the damaged lung will often heal.

If your baby regularly becomes short of oxygen after feeding, or after other activities , such as being bathed, she may also go home with temporary oxygen support.

When your baby is having oxygen therapy you need to keep a very careful eye on her if she has a respiratory infection. Ask your pediatrician about flu vaccine for her too and make sure that her whooping cough vaccination course is completed on time.

FEEDING YOUR BABY BY TUBE

Usually by the time a premature baby is well and strong enough to go home, she will be taking as much milk as she needs for herself, whether it is from your breast, from a bottle or from a special feeding cup (see page 116).

Some babies, however, are not able to do this just yet. This may be because they have heart or breathing disorders, a problem with their esophagus, because they still cannot quite manage to coordinate their sucking, breathing and swallowing, or because they get very tired before they finish their feeding. If a baby is not yet taking enough nourishment by nursing or drinking, she will also have her calorie levels regularly topped up with tube-feeding. Once babies have reached a certain size and are otherwise well enough, it may be possible for them to go home in spite of their need for tube feeding. Different NICUs have different policies as to how big is big enough to go home.

Using a nasogastric (NG) tube at home

If your baby is being fed in this way (see page 114), try to let her nurse on your breast or her bottle (if she is able to) as much as she can for the first part of the feeding. Then attach a small syringe filled with the rest of the bottled milk or with some of your own expressed milk that has been waiting warmed and ready next to you and feed it to your baby slowly by gravity flow.

Other forms of tube-feeding

Some babies cannot use an NG tube because it may block part of one of their nostrils and can make it more difficult to breathe. If so, an orogastric (OG) tube, which goes into the mouth, may be used instead. It is usually put in carefully before feeding and removed afterward each time. The removal and replacement of the OG tube can upset babies, however, and may make them gag or vomit.

HERNIAS

A hernia is a small loop of intestine that has managed to push its way through a weakness in the muscle of the baby's abdominal wall. It usually looks like a firm lump on the skin's smooth surface. Hernias are surprisingly common in premature babies, and will often disappear on their own. If a hernia appears in the baby's groin, it is known as an inguinal hernia, if it appears behind the baby's navel, it is an umbilical hernia.

Umbilical hernias tend to sort themselves out without any treatment, and have often vanished by the baby's first or second birthday. If it does not, the baby may have an operation to repair the small gap in the abdominal muscle wall. Inguinal hernias, which are far more common in boys, will often be repaired while babies are still on the NICU, as soon as the doctors are confident that they are mature enough to tolerate an anesthetic.

There is also a very small chance that any hernia may strangulate. This means it twists and cuts off its own blood supply. Signs of a strangulated hernia include the lump darkening or becoming bigger or tender to touch, vomiting and severe colicky pains.

If you see any of these signs, call your pediatrician right away, because if the hernia has indeed strangulated, it is a medical emergency. It can, however, be repaired very successfully with a prompt operation.

HELPING PREVENT SIDS

When a baby dies suddenly and no one can find the cause, this is called sudden infant death syndrome (SIDS) (also called "crib death"). Fortunately, SIDS is getting

Hernias in premature babies

★ Can affect up to one in four premature babies.

★ Are far more common in boys.

★ The less a baby weighs at birth or the more premature he is, the likelier he is to have one.

★ A hernia lump may appear to come and go. It can be especially noticeable if the baby is crying hard.

Trying to stop smoking

If you are a smoker, try to cut down, or better still give up altogether. Babies, especially premature babies, and cigarettes do not mix.

Unfortunately, giving up cigarettes is easy enough for health professionals and books to suggest but in the real world it can be very tough to do, because tobacco is so addictive. Also, you may never have felt more like smoking in your life. Having a premature baby can be very stressful, both when she is unwell and being cared for in the NICU and when she is back at home with you. But not smoking is such a vital part of keeping your baby healthy that it is worth trying hard to stop. (See *Helplines*, page 203).

Helping to protect your baby from SIDS

★ Put your baby on her back to sleep, unless your pediatrician instructs otherwise.

★ Ban smoking from your house. If you don't smoke and you don't let anyone else smoke anywhere near your baby, you reduce her risk of SIDS sevenfold.

★ Put your baby in the feet-to-foot sleep position—that is, with her feet right down at the end of the crib so she can't wriggle under her bedding and risk covering her head.

★ Do not put a pillow, stuffed toys, quilts or comforters in her crib—blankets and sheets are preferable. Do not use crib bumper pads.

★ Open a window—even just a crack—to allow fresh air into your baby's room.

★ If you are at all worried that your baby is not well, ask for help immediately. Health professionals give number one priority to premature babies who have recently come home. If you are worried that after repeated phone calls from you they may think you are a fussy parent, so be it. Being a fussy parent could save your baby's life.

★ Install a carbon monoxide alarm in your baby's bedroom, in addition to a working smoke alarm.

★ Use a firm crib mattress.

★ Do not let pets sleep in your baby's crib or bedroom.

increasingly rare. Within two years of the 1994 launch of the U.S. National Institute of Child Health & Human Development's "Back to Sleep" campaign—encouraging parents to place their babies on their backs or sides to sleep—the incidence of SIDS decreased by 30 percent. Similar campaigns in Canada and the U.K. have resulted in similar drops in the number of SIDS cases.

Parents of premature babies often worry about SIDS. Your baby was extremely well protected in the NICU where staff monitored her health continuously and were on hand immediately whenever there is a problem. Now that your baby is well and strong enough to go home with you, she will have her own much improved health and strength—and you—to help keep her safe and this will nearly always be all she needs. However, premature babies do run a higher risk of SIDS, and there are several important steps you can still take to protect them from this (now very small) possibility.

How warm should my baby be?

It is important to make sure that newborns and young babies do not get too hot, as that can increase the risk of SIDS. See pages 162–3 for advice on how warm you should keep your baby.

Sleep position

Putting newborns to sleep on their backs has vastly reduced (by as much as half) the incidence of SIDS and this may well be the safest position for your baby. However, the Foundation for the Study of Infant Deaths (FSID) says that for some premature babies—such as those who have particular types of breathing problem—this may not always be suitable. They advise talking to your neonatalogist or pediatrician about the best and most comfortable sleep position for your baby.

Alarms

If your baby's doctor advises you to let her sleep face down (prone), with her head to one side, and you are concerned about this, ask whether hiring or buying a baby alarm monitor (called an apnea/bradycardia alarm) for use at home would be helpful in your baby's case. There are two types:

one detects your baby's breathing pauses; the other goes off if her heartbeat becomes too slow. Either may be part of a sensor pad that the baby lies upon, or is attached around her middle with a special belt. Both are very different from the walkie-talkie style baby monitor devices where you leave one handset in your baby's room and take the other with you—these are just listening-in devices so you can hear your baby cry if you are in another part of the house.

However, these alarms may be more trouble than they are worth. Parents have reported being reduced to nervous wrecks by the number of frequent false alarms. One major survey in *Which?*, a major UK magazine, found that seven of every ten mothers gave up using the monitors because of this. Other parents say they became so dependent on the reassurance the monitor gave them they were afraid to go anywhere without it and so hardly ever went out at all.

It's important, too, to be aware that the alarms do not always detect trouble because sometimes they may not go off at all, or go off too late. For instance, though this is rare, if your baby's windpipe becomes blocked she may carry on making breathing movements and the alarm will not sound—but she can still suffocate. Another reported problem is that because the alarms have a preset time before they ring, they may not go off in time: though with a 20-second alarm, you do in practice have minutes in which to act, rather than seconds.

Breastfeeding

Premature babies are still extra vulnerable to catching bugs of all sorts for many months, even when they are well enough to go home, and infections are a risk factor in SIDS. Breastfeeding gives your baby extra protection against infections.

Firm crib mattress

No one has yet found a type of mattress that actually protects against SIDS. But it is best to use one that is firm, in good condition (get rid of it if it seems to be deteriorating), clean, dry and well aired. It is also recommended that babies should not have pillows, padded bumpers, extra linens or stuffed animals inside their cribs, because they might increase the risk of your baby overheating in bed.

"The monitor ruled our lives. It used to sound several times a day and each time my heart was in my mouth as I ran into her room. I found I could never relax, I kept expecting it to go off again any minute. But I would rather run to her a thousand times over for nothing than miss the one time when it was for real…"

Kim, father of Kirsty, born at 33 weeks

Emergency measures at home

If the alarm does go off, and you go quickly to your baby to find that she does need help, would you know what to do? Before you go home with your baby, ask her nurses to show you how to resuscitate her just in case you should ever need to; or, if you are already at home, ask your visiting nurse or doctor to show you.

173

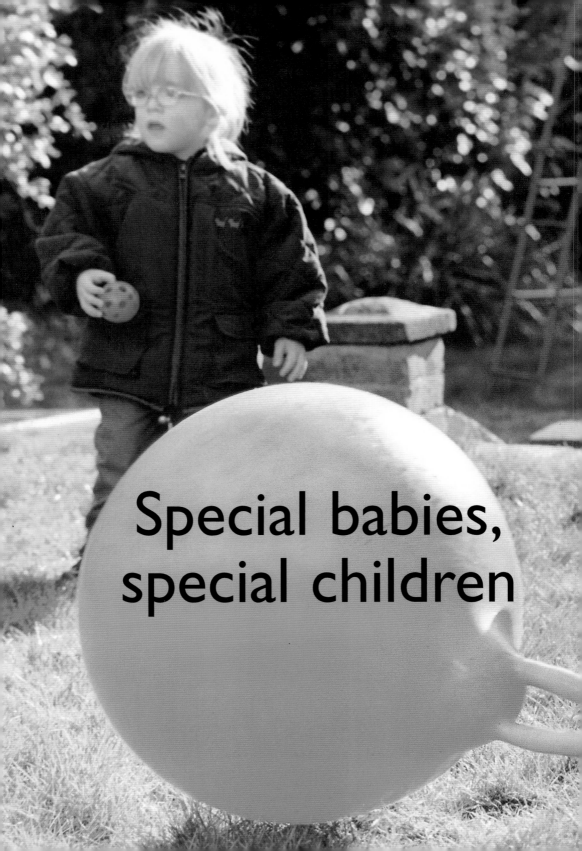

Special babies,
special children

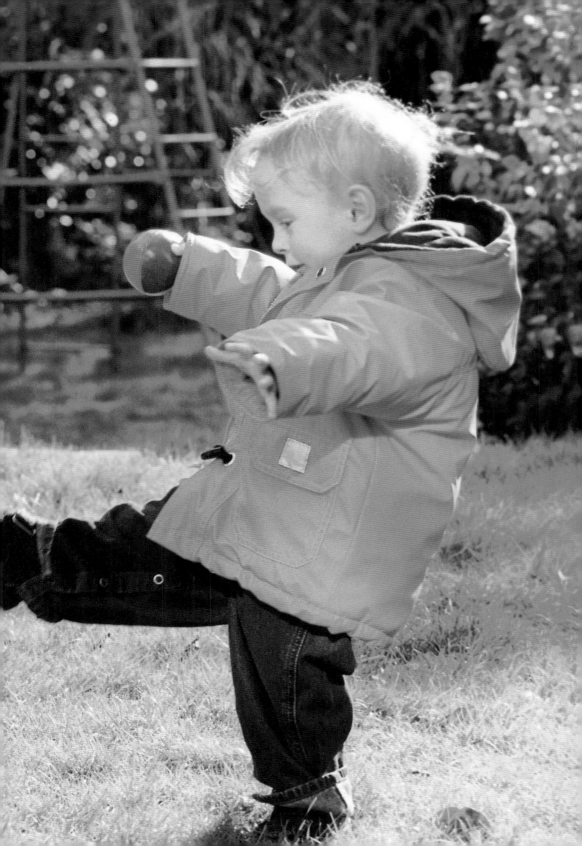

"We are very optimistic indeed about premature babies who are born from as little as 31 weeks. Most either have no ongoing problems at all, or if they do they tend to be very short-term."

Andrew Whitelaw, Professor of Neonatal Medicine at the University of Bristol, England and an international expert on the care and development of children born prematurely

"First it was a roller-coaster of: is he going to live? As he got better, it was: when can we take him home? Then, when we were all home, it was: how is he going to get on as he grows up? Is our son going to be normal? Now [at nine] he's already 4' 11", has his first two belts in karate, a wicked sense of humor, and is in the top of his class at school for everything except French..."

Mandy, whose son Christopher was born at 28 weeks, developed pneumonia then had a moderate IVH episode

Most premature babies now grow up fine, with no lasting physical or mental problems whatsoever. Research shows survival rates for babies of 31 weeks (gestational age) and over to be upward of 98 percent. In fact, overall, most babies born as early as 26 weeks will go on to do well.

Part of the reason for this is the now standard hospital practice of giving steroids to mothers who are in, or look as if they may begin, premature labor. This helps mature the lungs of their unborn babies while they are still in the uterus. More mature lungs mean easier breathing when a baby is born, and easier breathing means a better supply of oxygen to the brain. This is especially important because if the brain's supply of oxygen is interrupted or reduced, it can be damaged quite quickly. This damage may be very slight, but it can be substantial.

Another treatment that has improved premature babies' ability to breathe—and therefore their overall health and ability to survive without developing difficulties—is the practice of giving them surfactant replacement (see page 60).

Over the last two decades there have also been enormous improvements in high-tech life-support equipment for premature babies, such as sophisticated ventilator machines. In addition, there have been valuable advances in the methods of monitoring babies' blood pressure and blood oxygen levels, and huge improvements in the treatments for the types of problems premature babies are especially vulnerable to, from IVH and heart defects to infections.

POSSIBLE PROBLEMS

Most premature babies have no disabilities or ongoing difficulties at all. But it is also true that the earlier they were born, the more likely it is that they may have a problem. For most babies, the problem will either be a very mild one that is barely noticeable, such as squint, or a moderate difficulty, perhaps problems with coordinating movement, which will respond well to physiotherapy support and other treatments. But in a small number of cases, the disability may be more severe.

What is a disability?

Disability and handicap are words that are used very loosely. But in general they describe any physical or mental problem that prevents people from doing the things they would like to do for themselves, or which restricts the way they live.

Doctors divide disability into three grades: mild, moderate or severe. A severe disability means that the person needs physical help from someone else to manage his ordinary, everyday activities such as eating, washing, getting dressed or going out and about. Blindness, when someone can see nothing or only light or dark, profound deafness, severe cerebral palsy, and an IQ (see page 188) of below 70 points are all seen as potentially severe disabilities or handicaps.

Will my baby have a significant problem?

Professor Whitelaw estimates that the likelihood of a baby having a significant disability is about 10 percent if he was born at 28 weeks, and 20–30 percent if he was born very early, at around 24 or 25 weeks.

For four years a major British study, published in 1999, followed some 300 babies who were born extremely prematurely—that is, before 26 weeks. Results show that about half (51 percent) had no problems at all. A further quarter (26 percent) had mild to moderate problems, such as a hearing difficulty that could be corrected with a discreet hearing aid, short-sightedness that could be managed with the right pair of glasses, or a mild weakness in their legs that did not even interfere with their walking.

However, the remaining quarter (23 percent) of the children did have severe disabilities. These included significant cerebral palsy, major developmental delay, seizures, hydrocephalus that needed a permanent shunt (see page 72), and blindness.

Factors influencing the likelihood of disability

Apart from being born extremely early (before 26 weeks), there are also other factors that make it more likely that a baby might have a disability. If your child has experienced any of these, it makes good sense for him to have his sight

Risk factors for disability

These include:

★ Being born before 26 weeks

★ Becoming very short of oxygen while being born (birth asphyxia)

★ Bleeding in the brain (IVH)

★ Severe jaundice

★ Very low levels of sugar in the blood in the first few weeks of life (hypoglycemia)

★ Chronic, long-term illnesses (such as bronchopulmonary dysplasia)

★ Severe infections, such as those caused by herpes and Group B streptococcus

★ A long and difficult stay in a NICU

★ Having needed long-term ventilator support

The difference parents can make

"If a baby has a problem, parents can do a huge amount to help. I can still remember one particular little girl who was born prematurely and then had an intraventricular hemorrhage which all but devastated one side of her brain. But she was lucky enough to have terrific parents. Thanks to her mother, a Greek Cypriot, and her father, who was Polish, this little girl did so well that she was speaking three very different languages—English, Greek and Polish—by the time she was three.

"I have worked with several families like that, and have seen this happen again and again. This is why I know that parents' love, encouragement and stimulation can make such an enormous difference: because, at that age, a baby's brain is quite plastic. It can be very adaptable because it is constantly making so many new neurological connections while the child is still very young. So if one side is damaged, the other side can often take over."

Andrew Whitelaw, Professor of Neonatal Medicine at the University of Bristol

At almost three John is still very small, but he is growing up fast.

and hearing checked by hospital specialists before he leaves the NICU, and to have regular developmental check-ups afterward. This will help ensure that any problems will be noticed as early as possible. The sooner problems are detected, the more successful treatment and help will be.

A baby's home environment

A premature baby's home environment also has a great influence on the outcome of any problems. A good home environment has nothing whatever to do with wealth or privilege. It doesn't mean having a big, beautiful house or expensive toys. It means having loving, positive parents (or a parent) there who are consistently doing the best they can to encourage, care for and stimulate their baby in appropriate ways as he grows up. When a baby does have a good home environment, this can go a long way toward reducing the effects of many developmental problems.

Parents make a big difference

The impact of a baby's parents and his environment on his development cannot be emphasized enough, according to TrezMarie Zotkiewicz, Neonatal Discharge Coordinator at the Ochsner Foundation Hospital in New Orleans. "Infants with known developmental risks such as IVH may develop normally with early intervention and appropriate stimulation at home. Yet babies discharged as 'well' may return to follow-up clinics with significant delays, in part because of lack of learning opportunities at home." Most neonatal experts share this view.

FOLLOW-UP CARE: CHECKING AND SUPPORTING

When you go home with your premature baby, you need not feel alone. There are many health professionals and parents' help groups there to support you, and a big cast of specialists who can assess and help with your baby or child's development (see page 203).

Your baby's pediatrician will work with you to monitor your baby's progress after he leaves the NICU to go home with you, and address concerns you may have about his

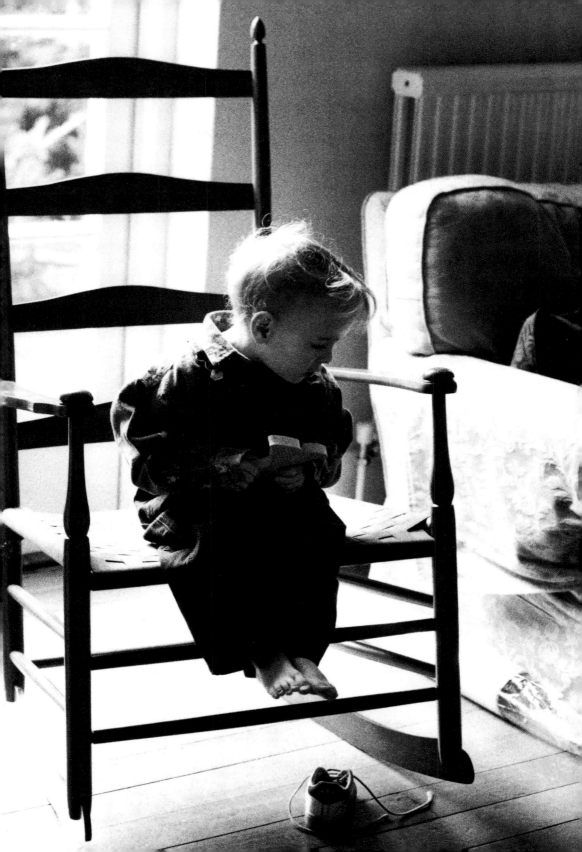

Worries

If you are worried about something, **you do not need to wait until the next check-up appointment** to discuss it. Call your pediatrician.

Variations in follow-up care

The schedule of follow-up visits given on these pages may vary from what you experience with your baby, depending on:

★ your baby's health

★ the NICU's program of care

★ your baby's doctors

★ where you live .

Remember that should you have any concerns, you should not hesitate to talk to your baby's doctor, one of the nurses you trust at the NICU, or your community health services.

health or development. Your baby's pediatrician may have to refer him to specialists, such as those in *Caring for your child* on page 203 whose job is to check your baby's developmental progress (his speech, hearing, movement and so on) and his physical and mental health at regular intervals, as he grows up into toddlerhood and beyond. If any difficulties arise, these specialists will help diagnose and treat them.

Parents say that it is very helpful and reassuring to develop a good relationship with their pediatrician, or a particular member of the doctor's or clinic's staff with whom you feel especially comfortable. This can make asking questions and mentioning any concerns you have much easier. It is also really important to go to every single follow-up appointment, whether it is a standard developmental check or a date with the audiologist to check your child's hearing.

Follow-up checks

Most follow-up visits for a baby who was born at 30 weeks or less will occur regularly until he is about two years old. If he has a particular problem, the appropriate specialist will keep an eye on his progress for longer, such as the respiratory pediatrician who would help your baby with breathing difficulties.

The timetable of your baby's check-ups will vary depending on the NICU hospital, local health authority practices, the specialists as well as on how well or unwell your child has been, on whether he has any particular problems and, if he does, on how severe these are. But the following is an example of the basic type of check-up schedule your child may have. Some of the stages depend on your baby's corrected age—his age counted from the day he would have been born if he had not arrived prematurely (see page 157).

The first visit One to two weeks after going home with your baby, you will visit your baby's pediatrician or, in some cases, the NICU's follow-up clinic. These visits can continue once or twice a week if you need them, for between six weeks and a year, depending on your child's needs and also on the hospital's policy and resources.

Six weeks (corrected age) Your baby will have his first assessment from his pediatrician, who will check your child's:

- movement and reflexes
- sight
- social development (Is he interested when you talk to him? Does he smile yet? Follow you about with his eyes?)
- hearing
- hips, as these may occasionally have been dislocated at birth
- weight, length and head size (its circumference)
- testes (if he is a boy) to see if these have descended (dropped) yet.

Immunizations Your doctor may also want to discuss immunizations with you. Most health professionals will prefer to give a premature baby the standard immunizations at the usual times, and will not take your baby's corrected age into account. The exception is the polio immunization which, as it is a live vaccine, will not be given when he is still in hospital.

Four months Your baby will have his first developmental check-up to assess neurological and general development. The four-month check is also a good chance to talk about anything at all that you may be worried about, however small it might be.

Seven months Your baby's neurological and general development will be checked and he will be given a hearing test.

Eight months The same things checked at six weeks will be checked again, for progress. As well, your baby will be checked as to what sorts of sounds he likes to make at the moment, as these are a prelude to learning to talk. Another hearing test may be done.

Twelve months A detailed assessment of your baby's development will be done. At this stage he may have other

Asking for specific information

Parents whose premature babies are now growing up say that it is helpful to try to get very specific answers to a few questions at every clinic visit—for example:

★ When will I know about x?

★ What does it mean if we see our child doing y?

★ How long will he need this therapy for?

★ When might we expect to see the therapy helping?

Then at least you will come away with some concrete information every time.

It can be very helpful to keep a notebook in which you can write questions down before you see the follow-up staff, and also to take notes of their answers.

"If your baby was born prematurely, try to learn what is normal for your particular child and to treat him as normal; no two children, whether they were born very early or at term, ever develop at exactly the same rate.

Just expect to need to 're-frame' things from time to time. Re-framing means re-evaluating what to expect from your child as he grows up, each time he makes another stride forward, or each time you have another piece of news about a particular aspect of his development from the clinic. Parents say this re-framing is a continuous process."

Chrissie Israel, Parent-Baby Interaction Advisor at Southmead Hospital, Bristol

appointments or be referred to a specialist, depending on whether or not any particular problems—perhaps with hearing, vision, movement, or feeding—have come up.

Twelve to eighteen months A developmental check will be done on all the things looked at before, to ascertain your baby's progress, as well as his speech will be checked.

Three and a half years Your child may be given a preschool development assessment.

YOUR CHILD'S DEVELOPMENT

Neonatal experts and parents whose premature babies are growing up into toddlerhood and beyond all say that it is best not to expect a smooth, textbook development. All babies have their own individual timetables for doing things, and this is especially so for premature babies. Long-term illness, a difficult stay in hospital, an ongoing health problem or a disability are all things that may slow down your baby's progress.

It is hard not to make comparisons with other children who were born at term, or when reading baby-and-childcare books, but try to bear in mind two important things: your child's corrected age and the fact that most premature babies do "catch up," but in their own time. Parents say it is very encouraging to keep a diary of all your child's steps forward and achievements and that sometimes when thay look back at it, they are amazed and comforted by how far their children have come.

Growth

A child's growth is affected by many different things. These include how well he is, how much he weighed when he was born, how early he was born, genetics (the things he inherits from you, his parents), whether he needed special care at an NICU, of what sort and how long he stayed. Other important factors include the sort of health problems your child has had so far, how he was cared for in hospital, and how he is looked after at home.

Babies weighing more than 2 pounds 3 ounces (1000g) at birth will usually have more or less caught up by the time they are four or five years old. But, babies born weighing less will take longer to reach their growth potential (that is, the best growth they can achieve). However, with the high-calorie milk formulas now available, most babies who were born prematurely are now reaching their growth potential faster than they did ten years ago.

Action Keep an eye on your child's weight and height using the standard growth charts at your doctor's office or the NICU might give you one when your baby goes home. If you have any concerns at all, for example worries about feeding difficulties, either your pediatrician, nurse practitioner or the staff at your baby's clinic can help advise and support you.

Parents are often worried about whether their child is growing properly. "Try to look at the rate at which he is growing, rather than how big he is," suggests Neil Marlow, Professor of Neonatal Medicine at Nottingham University. "If a child is growing at a normal rate, then he is probably fine, even if he is smaller than other children of his age who were born at term."

If he is not growing at a normal rate, contact your pediatrician. He or she will probably want to examine your child carefully and perhaps carry out some tests to see if there is any reason for this. It is not likely that a specialist would give your child treatment with growth hormone these days, despite the amount of press coverage it has had over the years. This is because, according to Professor Marlow, the gain in height that it gives is only short term.

Sight

Around a quarter of babies born weighing less than 2 pounds 3 ounces (1000g) will have some sort of difficulty with their sight, but for babies weighing more, this drops sharply to just 2 percent.

One of the vision problems that often affects very premature babies is retinopathy of prematurity or ROP (see page 74). In its most severe form this can cause blindness. According to Anthony Kaiser, Neonatologist at St. Thomas's Hospital in London, ROP affects around one third of babies born before 28 weeks. Eight out of ten

Premature babies who were born at 34 weeks or later and were the right weight for the amount of time they have spent in the uterus (doctors may use the term *appropriate for gestational age*, or *AGA* to describe this) will usually grow at around the same rate as a term baby.

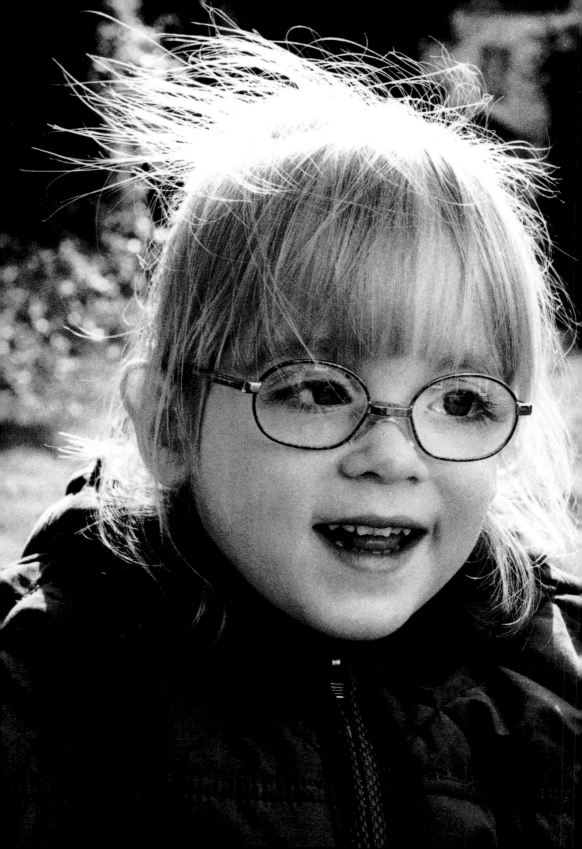

babies who develop the condition do so only mildly and it sorts itself out with no treatment at all.

The most common problems are far less serious. They include a mild to moderate squint and near- or far-sightedness, which can be corrected with the right pair of glasses.

Action All premature babies should be examined by an ophthalmologist, preferably before they leave the NICU to go home, or at any rate when they are around six weeks old, and at regular intervals after that until the blood vessels of their eyes have matured. If there are any signs of ROP they can be watched closely, and if necessary treated with gentle laser therapy. In some areas, your baby will also routinely have sight checks for squints, short sight and long sight when he is one year old.

Hearing

Some studies suggest that more than one in 10 premature babies (about 13 percent) may have some form of hearing loss, compared with one in 50 babies born at term. Hearing problems are more likely if babies were born extremely prematurely, because their hearing systems are still maturing as late as 24–26 weeks and might still be especially vulnerable to damage if they have to complete the process outside the protection of the uterus.

One possible additional cause of hearing damage in premature babies is the surprising amount of noise they are exposed to in the NICU. Research suggests an incubator can be a very noisy place, with sound levels reaching between 50 and 90 decibels (dB). In an ordinary home, the level is nearer 40 dB. Other risk factors include IVH (see page 70), shortage of oxygen at birth, severe jaundice, some infections including bacterial meningitis, and a birth weight of less than 3 pounds 5 ounces (1500g).

Action Hearing difficulties can make it harder for a child not only to listen to language but also to speak clearly himself, so it can have a secondary effect on learning and behavior. If they cannot hear properly, children may become thoroughly discouraged and so withdraw. They may also appear to be disobedient, or behave aggressively

"Overall, premature babies tend to grow up to be fairly slim and light in their earlier years.

"It is normal for their growth to be between the 10th and 25th percentile on the growth chart; the average term baby's growth is usually somewhere near the middle on the 50th percentile.

"But, as teenagers, they usually finish up only about an inch shorter than you would have expected them to be by looking at their parents' heights."

Neil Marlow, Professor of Neonatal Medicine, Nottingham University

Born at 27 weeks, Emily Grace is now a bright and healthy three-year-old, the only remaining signs of her prematurity being a degree of far-sightedness easily corrected with glasses, and a squint which will be cured by an operation when she is a little older.

Breathing

Please see *Time to go home*, pages 168–70 on possible breathing problems and coming home with oxygen.

or disruptively out of sheer frustration, so it vital to detect any hearing difficulties as early as possible.

If a baby was born prematurely, especially if he has any of the above risk factors, he needs to be screened by an audiologist before he goes home from the NICU, then again three to six months later. This will help make sure that, if there is a problem of any sort, it will be diagnosed early, then treated promptly and effectively.

Speech

At around the age of two, as many as 20 to 40 percent of toddlers who were born prematurely, especially those born at less than 2 pounds 3 ounces (1000g), may have some difficulty with language. If they do have a language problem they often find it easier to understand what is said to them than they do to express themselves with words.

These children usually have normal or above average IQs, so this difficulty with language is not something that is directly linked with their intelligence.

Action It is enormously helpful to talk to your child a great deal from the very beginning, even if you think he is too young to understand. Keep an eye on the way your toddler communicates with you, whether he is trying to imitate words, and whether he is succeeding with any, and if you have any concerns at all, let your baby's pediatrician know. He or she can always refer your child for a check-up (and for extra help if it is needed) with a speech therapist.

Language abilities

Ideally, a toddler needs to be able to:

★ Respond to simple instructions ("Please give me the ball," or "Come over here to me") by the time he is about 18 months corrected age.

★ Put two words together by about two years corrected age.

★ Speak a few words that someone who didn't know the child could understand by about two and a half years corrected age.

★ Speak in simple sentences of more than two or three words by the time he is about three (corrected age).

Movement

It is fairly common for babies who were born prematurely to have a degree of "unusual muscle tone" for their first year or so of life. In fact, at least 40 percent—and possibly as much as 80 percent—of those born weighing less than 3½ pounds (1600g) have this to some extent. Their leg or arm muscles may be stiffer or floppier than usual, their movements may be a bit jerky, and they may have exaggerated or muted muscle reflexes too. However, these things generally sort themselves out without any treatment at all by the time the children are 12–18 months old.

For some infants however, the abnormal muscle tone does not sort itself out and they may be diagnosed as having a degree of cerebral palsy (CP). Doctors define this as "abnormal posture or movement which has been caused by damage to part of the brain." In practice, this may mean that a person's muscles are very stiff or even in spasm, which can be painful, or they may be very floppy. Both muscle stiffness and floppiness make it hard to sit, stand, walk or control movement.

Risk factors that make it more likely that a baby may have cerebral palsy include: shortage of oxygen in the uterus, at birth or for the first few days afterward; being born very prematurely; and severe IVH. The types of difficulties a child experiences if he has CP may depend on which area of his brain was damaged, and how mild or severe that damage is.

What parents may notice first Children with cerebral palsy may find it difficult to reach the usual milestones you would expect to see in a baby or toddler's development, such as sitting, crawling, walking and balancing, reaching out for objects, grasping small things and beginning to make smaller and more precise movements such as coloring and scribbling with crayons. They may also have trouble with their speech, and difficulty eating. Physical symptoms can include joint stiffness, turned out ankles, scoliosis (where the spine leans or twists sideways) or a dislocated hip. Children with cerebral palsy often have IQs that are either normal or above average, but despite this they may experience some learning difficulties too.

Action If your baby is diagnosed as having "abnormal muscle and/or reflexes" this does not necessarily mean he has cerebral palsy. Only three to six percent of premature babies have true CP and many of these children have only a mild form. What it does mean is that your pediatrician and specialists will help you monitor his progress until a clearer picture emerges. A physiotherapist or occupational therapist may show you some special gentle exercises for you to help your child do, and other activities to help his muscle and ligament development.

"Many of the early milestones in a child's development are movement milestones: the age at which they roll over, sit up, crawl, or walk. For many extremely preterm babies these milestones will just arrive late, along with other areas of their development. But most babies do simply catch up later."

Ros Jones, consultant neonatologist at Wrexham Park Hospital, Slough

Cerebral palsy (CP)

CP can be very mild, moderate or severe. It can also be difficult to diagnose accurately at first. However, the more severely affected a baby is, the more quickly he can be diagnosed, and the more quickly he can be helped (see page 78).

"The doctors said Andy may have cerebral palsy but that they would not be able to tell for sure until he was about a year and a half old. We thought: how can we possibly wait that long to find out? He's a year now, he still has some muscle stiffness but still no one can give us a clear answer. But Andy is a lovely little boy—and what's more, he's ours. We just want to enjoy our son for who he is; we're not going to get obsessed about what might be wrong. We don't want to put a label on him. We'll just see how this all turns out."

Judith, mother of Andrew, born at 29 weeks

IQ

IQ, meaning Intelligence Quotient, is one basic and useful measure of intelligence.

"Average intelligence" is considered to be anything over 85 points. Below-average (sometimes called below-normal or sub-normal) intelligence is considered to be 70–84 points.

Any observations or changes that mothers and fathers see may provide the most important clues or early warning systems of all. You know your own child best so mention any concerns you have, or any changes you notice.

If your child does have cerebral palsy rather than the type of different muscle tone that disappears after 12–18 months, physiotherapy, regular gentle exercises and stretching can help. Special braces can provide support, and surgery may also, if needed, be used later on to help straighten his limbs.

There is also a good deal of research and experimental work being tried to find other forms of treatment, including using small doses of a substance called botulism toxin. This is a poison, but research at the Walton Centre for Neurology and Neurosurgery in Liverpool suggests that, used carefully, it may relax the painful muscle spasms of cerebral palsy and improve a child's posture and walking, possibly delaying or even in some cases avoiding the need for operations .

For a list of organizations that may be able to help you, please see page 203.

Learning and IQ

The vast majority of children who were born prematurely have a perfectly normal IQ, or an IQ that is above average. Research in the early 1990s found that of very low birthweight premature babies, around two-thirds had IQs of between 85 and 115 (average intelligence). Another one-quarter (20–24 percent) had borderline IQs of between 75 and 85 and about one in 20 (5 percent) had an IQ rating of less than 70.

Babies who were born very prematurely or who had very low birthweights of below 2 pounds 3 ounces (1000g) have a greater risk of having a problem than babies born less prematurely and weighing more than this. Estimates vary, but one large research study found that about one in ten (8–13 percent) of babies born weighing less than 2 pounds 3 ounces (1000g) had below normal IQ levels. But this also means that nine out of ten of the babies had perfectly normal or even higher than average IQs.

For extremely small premature babies weighing less than 1 pound 10 ounces (750g) at birth, four out of every five had perfectly normal IQ levels, with one in five (20 percent) having below average IQ.

Action Regular developmental assessments with specialists are very important. Keep an eye on your child's progress. If anything worries you at all, or just does not seem quite right, do not let it go. Talk to your baby's pediatrician or other specialists and speaking with other mothers of premature babies who may have experienced something similar with their own children is also very helpful.

Try to give your child as much loving support and appropriate stimulation as you can—while still letting him

Happy and confident, facing the world

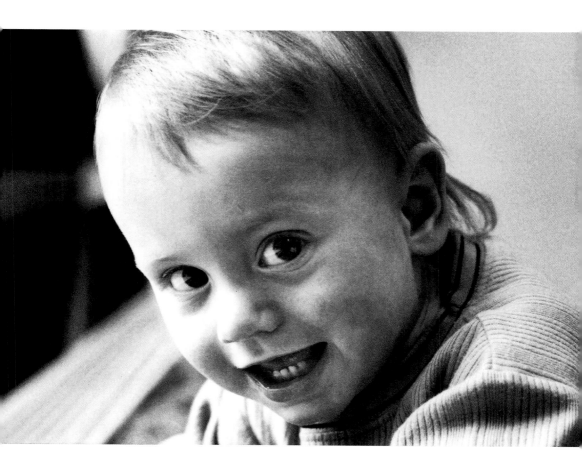

develop at his own pace. This just might not be the same pace as children who were born at term, especially if he has had a difficult start or has a long-term health problem he is trying to cope with or overcome. If you are worried about his progress, ask your child's school board what extra learning programs may be available to help his development.

Learning and behavior

As with other developmental problems, the later a baby was born, the milder and fewer his difficulties are likely to be—but the earlier he was born, the more problems he may have at school.

Starting school Ideally, a school should take your child's corrected age into account, especially if he was born as much as three or four months prematurely (at 24–28 weeks). Your child may not be quite ready to start full-time school at the "standard" age, particularly if your school board requires children to join the pre-kindergarten classes when they are four. Unfortunately, not all school principals may be sympathetic to this idea and, even if they are, they may not be able to help if, as is quite usual, the school board has strict rules (sometimes based on funding criteria) about when a child must start. But it is worth asking, because at the very least you may be able to get the principal to allow your child just to come for mornings only for a couple of terms if he finds full days too a bit much to cope with.

Possible problems According to studies, attention deficit disorder or ADD (short concentration span, impulsiveness) and hyperactivity are about four to five times more common for babies who were born weighing less than 3 pounds 5 ounces (1500g). In any group of small boys and girls, up to 6 percent might have some degree of either ADD or hyperactivity anyway; however, for children who arrived prematurely some studies put it nearer to 25 percent.

At the other end of the behavioral spectrum, parents, researchers and teachers also say they have noticed that some children born very prematurely who weighed less than 2 pounds 3 ounces (1000g) at birth are more likely to be quite shy, withdrawn and nervous of being assertive or standing up for themselves at school.

Even when premature children have perfectly normal or above average intelligence ratings—as many do—they also seem to be more likely than term-born children to have difficulties with their school work. Possible problem areas include reading, spelling, math, abstract reasoning, and difficulty organizing themselves and their work. So extra help at school is still much needed and can make a great deal of difference.

Long-term research that followed up premature children for several years through school up to the ages of nine, ten and eleven has found that there may be "residual" learning problems. These are difficulties that are not obvious at first, and that are only noticed by parents and teachers as the children become older. The problems may be quite subtle and sometimes go unrecognized for several school years. However, the children tend not to outgrow them on their own, so they may need extra help.

The good news is that only around 10–20 percent of children who were very low birthweight premature babies and who have normal intelligence have any kind of learning disability that is marked enough for it to affect how they do at school.

Action Understanding, encouragement and support from both parents and teachers are vital. Try to identify any areas in which your child is having difficulty at school as early as possible, ensuring he has special long-term help and support there from the beginning.

If a child is fairly quiet, is seen to be getting on with things, makes little fuss, and has no very obvious difficulties with, for example, reading or writing, teachers with big classes to cope with may assume he is doing fine when in fact he may be struggling. This can go on for years before anyone notices.

If you are concerned because you feel your child needs some extra support at school, but his teacher is not convinced, talk to the pediatrician. He or she will often be able to support you by writing letters to the school, and referring your child for assessment and help to the right community education support services and specialists, such as an educational psychologist.

Regular checks on your child's sight and hearing are important, too, as even minor problems can make a great difference to his understanding of what is going on in the classroom and playground.

As your child gets older (from about four or five) see what extracurricular activities he is interested in as these may well help to build up his confidence in himself. Parents often mention that some of the most helpful things for gentle confidence building include drama, art, music or dance classes, swimming, martial arts, and the special yoga/meditation classes for children that are available in some areas.

If your child does have a learning disability, whether it is very mild or more serious, it's well worth contacting a parent and family support group (see page 203). These organizations can offer all sorts of help, including moral support and information about everything from the type of diet and nutritional supplements that may help, to special forms of education and how to get educational back-up, such as special classes or tutoring.

PREMATURE BIRTH: WHY DOES IT HAPPEN?

Perhaps one of the hardest things about having a premature baby is that in one case out of every two, no one can even tell you why it happened. However, parents do often wonder whether there was any reason for their child's early birth, or whether there is any treatment the doctors could give, or some steps they can take for themselves, that might help prevent another premature birth next time.

It's not your fault

Many women feel that if they have a premature baby it must somehow be their fault. Experts say that is very rarely true. On the contrary, they say that women who give birth early have usually done a terrific job of protecting and nurturing their babies under very difficult circumstances.

REASONS FOR PREMATURITY

There are two ways in which babies may be born too soon. One is if their mothers go into labor too early. This is called *premature labor*. Or, there may be a medical problem threatening the well-being of the unborn baby, her mother or sometimes both, and the obstetrician may arrange to deliver the baby early. This is called *premature delivery*.

Causes of premature labor

There are many different reasons for giving birth early, several of which are inter-related. The main causes seem to be:

• **An infection** around the cervix, or in the uterus. Other infections, notably those of the kidneys and urinary system, are also sometimes associated with early labor.

• A **"sensitive" uterus** that can easily be provoked to contract strongly and much earlier than normal, especially if overly stretched by a big baby or twins or more.

• **Other problems with the uterus**, such as placental abruption (when the placenta begins to peel away from the uterine wall). If there is any bleeding from behind the placenta this may irritate the muscle of the uterus and cause early contractions.

• **A weak cervix**, not strong enough to stay closed against the baby's increasing weight.

• **The baby not growing properly**, often because the placenta is not able to transmit enough food and oxygen. Pre-eclampsia (see below) can be a major cause of this.

• **Amniotic sac membranes that begin to weaken or give way early** (your waters breaking early).

• **Carrying twins, triplets or more** can stretch the uterus more than just one baby, and it also means extra weight is pressing down on the cervix, which may make it harder for it to remain shut.

• **An unusually shaped uterus; or a uterus that has a fibroid or fibroids** growing on its walls. Fibroids are benign, non-cancerous whorls of tissue.

• **Too much fluid in the amniotic sac** can put extra pressure on the walls of the uterus and perhaps the cervix too.

• **An abnormality in the fetus**. The mother's body may recognize that an unborn fetus is not developing normally and end the pregnancy by going into early labor. This usually happens in the first 12 weeks, as a miscarriage, but occasionally it may occur later, as a premature birth.

• **Physical trauma**, such as an accident, fall, violence or injury to the woman's belly.

• **Rogue antibodies** that cause blood clotting in the system. The condition is called thrombophilia.

• **"Placental clock" theory** Recent Australian research suggests that if unborn babies are not getting enough food and oxygen, they may be preprogrammed with a survival instinct that causes them to trigger labor—on the grounds that they might be "better out than in."

Other causes

There are many, and several of them are interrelated. Yet, as James McGregor, Professor of Obstetrics and Gynecology at Colorado University, says: "Premature birth is like heart disease in a way—there are so many different risk factors. And why is it that some mothers with major risk factors don't have their babies prematurely, yet others, with no major risk factors that we can see, do? We still have no idea."

• **Having diabetes**—or developing it temporarily while you are pregnant. Diabetes is a risk factor for developing pre-eclampsia. So are other long-term health problems such as high blood pressure and kidney disease.

• **Smoking cigarettes.**

• **Continuously high stress levels.**

• **Being poor.**

• **Heavy drinking** and/or binge drinking.

• **Heavy physical work**, constant standing, heavy lifting, and so on.

• **Taking illegal recreational drugs**. For instance, if you smoke cannabis regularly, research suggests you are more likely to have a low-birthweight baby (low-birthweight babies have many of the same difficulties as premature babies); cocaine and crack may also be risk factors for having a premature baby, partly because they cause blood pressure swings, which may encourage placental abruption.

• **Being an underweight mother.**

• **Being an "older" mother (over 35) or a much younger one (under 17).** It is possible that as you get older, if you do develop pre-eclampsia you may do so more severely. You may also be likely to develop temporary (gestational) diabetes.

• **Infections** causing very high temperatures can trigger premature labor.

• **Becoming pregnant through assisted conception techniques** such as IVF may be a risk factor insofar as it makes multiple pregnancy more likely. However, it tends to be older women who have this type of fertility treatment, and their likelihood of a premature baby may be higher anyway.

• **Work.** There is no proof that working, as such, when you are pregnant makes you more likely to have a premature baby. However, according to a large European study (EUROPOP '98), in addition to heavy manual labor, there are some particular types or aspects of work that may make a difference. These include jobs that cause continual stress and working long hours (43 hours or more a week).

Premature delivery

There are various reasons why your doctors may decide it is safest to deliver your baby early.

• **Pre-eclampsia**, a pregnancy-related form of high blood pressure (*note*: raised blood pressure in pregnancy is not uncommon and does not, by itself, mean you have pre-eclampsia). Symptoms include headaches and swelling or puffiness in your hands, feet, legs and sometimes face. It can be detected by regular antenatal checks: signs include raised blood-pressure readings and protein traces in the urine. Pre-eclampsia is most common in first pregnancies and is usually mild, but about one in every hundred women who develop it do so severely. It starts in the placenta, reducing the mother's blood flow and so cutting back the baby's source of nutrition and oxygen. This means the baby will not grow very well, or stop growing altogether or, in extreme cases, may die.

• **Problems with the placenta** can mean your unborn baby is undernourished and not growing properly, so your doctors may feel it would be better if she were delivered early and given the best possible care, and nutrition, in the NICU. Other problems include placenta praevia (where the placenta is blocking the baby's exit route).

• **Carrying twins, triplets or more**. Your doctors may decide it is safer to deliver them early if perhaps one, or more, of them does not seem to be growing in the uterus, or if you are finding being pregnant with more than one baby very difficult.

• "**Maternal reasons**" means that the mother needs an early delivery as she is unable to cope with the pregnancy any longer. For example, she may have severe pain because her pubic bones have separated or may have had troubled previous pregnancies, or a previous pregnancy that ended in stillbirth.

WHAT ABOUT NEXT TIME?

If you have had one premature baby, it is true that you are more likely than a mother whose last baby arrived at term to have another. However, doctors will monitor both your own and your baby's health more closely than the first time around so that they can identify and help treat any problems quickly and effectively.

What can you do?

If you are a smoker, try your very best to stop before you become pregnant again, or at the very least, as soon as you know you are pregnant (see page 203 for sources of help and support). Smoking when you are pregnant means that your baby may be born earlier—but it also means that your baby will almost certainly be born smaller, because smoking restricts the food and oxygen she gets in the uterus, and retards growth, so she will be more likely to be low birthweight and have many of the same difficulties as premature babies.

If you are taking illegal drugs, try to get as much help as you can to give them up, if possible before you become pregnant again.

Try to cut down your stress levels in any way you can, and eat and drink as healthily as possible. Some doctors recommend cutting out alcohol altogether; however, there is some evidence that a single glass of red wine a day may do no harm, as red wine contains ingredients that help prevent damage to blood vessels, including those in the placenta. Consult with your doctor if you have concerns.

If you had your baby early last time and no one knows why, it is worth asking your hospital to do a simple swab test to check for an infection in your vagina or cervix. Infections in the cervix can be low-level, produce no symptoms, and live undetected for many years yet still be an important cause of premature labor.

Preventing premature birth

- **Pre-eclampsia**. If you had pre-eclampsia last time, especially if it began before you were 32 weeks pregnant, your doctors may suggest a daily low dose of aspirin (usually 75mg or one-quarter of one adult tablet), beginning when you are about 12 weeks pregnant. Aspirin reduces the blood-clotting chemicals your body makes, and might also discourage your blood vessels from contracting. However, low-dose aspirin is not a self-help treatment: it needs to be taken under the supervision of a doctor.

You will be given frequent and detailed antenatal check-ups throughout your pregnancy to look out for any signs of pre-eclampsia beginning again. These include urine and blood-pressure checks, scans to track your baby's growth and Doppler scans to check the blood flow through the placenta. The obstetrician may advise bed rest, and might give you medication to keep your blood pressure down. If the pre-eclampsia is making you ill, or it looks as if you may be going into premature labor, you will be admitted to hospital for careful monitoring, bed rest, and possibly drugs to lower your blood pressure.

Recent research suggests that vitamins C and E taken in the last half of your pregnancy can help prevent from pre-eclampsia developing.

- **Weak cervix**. A surgical stitch may help keep the cervix closed: a study by the Royal College of Gynaecologists found it could work for anything between 1 and 19 weeks, and seemed to help in 50 percent of cases.
- **Thrombophilia** is relatively rare, though it is more common for women who have an autoimmune disorder called lupus. It can be treated with medications that reduce blood clotting.
- **When the baby is not growing properly**. If this is due to high blood pressure you will be offered drugs to lower it, advised to rest in bed (perhaps in hospital) and be carefully monitored. If your baby's growth seems very restricted, and/or she seems to be in distress, your obstetrician may decide to deliver her and give her the best possible care in the NICU.

Treatments for premature labor

If you are in premature labor already, or if your waters have broken but you have no contractions yet, you may be given antibiotics to treat existing infections or prevent one from developing. This treatment is still experimental, but it may help because it is thought that infections produce inflammatory substances that trigger labor.

When labor has started

You will be admitted to hospital, monitored carefully, given bed rest and probably offered a drug treatment that can delay premature labor, because unless your baby is in distress (perhaps she is short of oxygen, now) every extra day she spends inside you counts.

A couple of extra days or so make the most difference at around the 26–27 week mark when, American research suggests, an unborn baby is maturing especially quickly and her chances of survival rise by around 1 percent for every extra 24 hours she is able to spend in the uterus. Buying a further 24–48 hours also gives your obstetrician vital time to make sure that there is a guaranteed place waiting for her in a good neonatal care unit as soon as she arrives.

Research, medical studies and resources

EFFECTS OF PREMATURITY; CARE OF AND INTERACTION WITH PREMATURE BABIES

Type of handling your baby receives

American Academy of Pediatrics. *Guidelines for Perinatal Care*. Elk Grove Village, Illinois: American Academy of Pediatrics, 1992.

Werner, N. P. and A. E. Conway. Caregiver contacts experienced by premature infants in neonatal intensive care. *Maternal-Child Nursing Journal* 19(11):21–43, 1990.

Lighting levels in NICUs

Glass, P., et al. Effect of bright light in the hospital nursery on the incidence of retinopathy of prematurity. *New England Journal of Medicine*, 313(7):401–404, 1985.

Lotas, M. J. Effects of light and sound in the neonatal intensive care unit environment in the low birth weight infant. *Clinical Issues in Perinatal and Women's Health Nursing* 3(1):34–44, 1992.

Oehler, J. M. Developmental care of low birthweight infants. *Nursing Clinics of North America* 28(2):289–301, 1993.

Robinson J., et al. Illuminance of neonatal units. *Archives of Diseases in Childhood* 65:679–682, 1990.

Whitley, S., and M. Cowan. Developmental intervention in the newborn intensive care unit. *NAACO's Clinical Issues in Perinatal and Women's Health Nursing* 2(1):84–110, 1991.

Babies sleeping only for brief periods

Korones, S. B. Disturbance and infants' rest. In *Report on the 69th Ross Conference on Pediatric Research* edited by T. D. Moore. Columbus: Ross Laboratories, 1976

Premature baby massage

Field, T. M. Tactile/kinesthetic stimulation effects on preterm neonates. *Pediatrics* 77:654–658, 1986.

Johnson & Johnson Pediatric Round Table. Effect of touch on the immune system. In *Advances in Touch* edited by N. Gunzenhauser, 14:22031, 1989.

Kuhn, C., et al. Tactile/kinesthetic stimulation effects on sympathetic and adrenocortical function in preterm infants. *Journal of Pediatrics*: 119, 1991.

Therapeutic touch

Carruthers, A. Therapeutic touch: a force to promote bonding and wellbeing. *Professional Nurse* Feb. 1992.

Daley, B. Therapeutic touch: nursing practice and contemporary cutaneous wound healing research. *Journal of Advanced Nursing* 25:1123–1132, 1997.

Fedoruk, R. B. Therapeutic touch as a method for reduction of stress in premature neonates. Dissertation in *Abstracts International* 46, 1984.

Olsen, M., et al. Stress induced immunosuppression and therapeutic touch. *Alternative Therapies* 3(2):68–74, 1997.

Quinn, J. F. *Transfer of the Relaxation Response*. Doctoral dissertation, University of Maryland, Maryland. (Also in *Journal of Holistic Nursing* 6(1), 1988.)

Meehan, T. C. Therapeutic touch and post-operative pain: a Rogerian research study *Nursing Science Quarterly* 6(2): pages 69–78, 1993.

Positioning of baby

Amiel-Tyson, C., and A. Grenier. *Neurological Assessment in the First Year of Life*. New York: Oxford University Press, 1986.

Blackburn, Susan. Problems of preterm infants after discharge. *Journal of Obstetric, Gynecologic, and Neonatal Nursing* 24:43–49, Jan. 1995.

Hallsworth, M. Positioning of the preterm infant. *Paediatric Nursing*, 7(1):18–20, 1995.

Turrill, S., and M. Stein. Supported positioning in intensive care. *Paediatric Nursing* 4(4), 1992.

Young, J. Nursing preterm babies in intensive care. Which position is best? *Journal of Neonatal Nursing* 1(1):27–31, 1994.

Position premature babies lie in affecting their postural development

Hallsworth, M. Positioning of the preterm infant. *Paediatric Nursing*, 7(1):18–20, 1995.

Young, J. Nursing preterm babies in intensive care. Which position is best? *Journal of Neonatal Nursing* 1(1):27–31, 1994.

Positioning/less medication

Jorgensen, K.M. *Developmental Care of the Premature Infant: A Concise Overview*. S. Weymouth: Developmental Care Division of Children's Medical Ventures, 1993.

Merenstein, G. B., and S. L. Gardner. *The Handbook of Neonatal Intensive Care*, 3rd ed. St. Louis: Mosby Year Book, 1993.

Kangaroo care

Hosseini, R. B., et al. Pre-term infants and fathers: psychological and behavioural effects of skin-to-skin contact. *Ursus Medicus* 2:47–55, 1992.

Ludington-Hoe, Susan, with Susan K. Golant. *Kangaroo Care: The Best You Can Do To Help Your Preterm Infant*. New York: Bantam, 1996.

——— and G.C. Anderson. Preliminary results of very early kangaroo care for preterm infants. Paper presented at 8th National Meeting of the Nurses' Association of the American College of Obstetricians & Gynecologists, Orlando, 1991.

——— and F. Hashemia. Temporal relationship between kangaroo care and crying. Paper presented at the International Sigma Theta Tau Meeting, Nov. 1991.

Virgin, C. The kangaroo method brings the child back to its mother. *Sygeplejersken* 11, 1987.

Whitelaw, A., et al. Skin to skin contact for very low birthweight infants and their mothers: a randomized trial of kangaroo care. *Archives of Diseases in Childhood* 63:1377–81, 1988.

Born smiling

Leboyer, Frederick. *Birth Without Violence*. London: Cedar Press, 1995.

Doing what, when: term and preterm babies

Gomez, Joan. *Childhood Development*. London: Vermilion, 1997.

Manginello, Frank, and Theresa Foy DiGeronimo. *Your Premature Baby*.

Chichester, West Sussex: John Wiley, 1991.

Volpe, Joseph J. *Neurology of the Newborn.* 2nd ed. Philadelphia: W.B. Saunders, 1987.

Premature survival rates

Tin, W., et al. Changing prognosis for babies of less than 28 weeks gestation. *British Medical Journal* 314: 107–11, 1997.

Morrison, J. Clinical, scientific and ethical aspects of fetal and neonatal care at extremely preterm periods of gestation. *British Journal of Obstetrics & Gynaecology* 104:1431–1350, Dec. 1997.

Unborn babies, awareness in uterus

Bradford, Nikki. *The Miraculous World of Your Unborn Baby.* London: Bramley Books, 1998.

Busnel, Marie, et al. Fetal audition. Annals of New Yord Academy of Sciences 662: 118–134, 1992.

Chamberlain, David. *The Mind of Your Newborn Baby.* Berkeley, California: North Atlantic Books, 1998.

Stenneert, E., et al. Incubator noise and hearing loss. *Early Human Development* 1(1):113–115.

Van de Carr, Rene, et al. Effects of a prenatal intervention programme. In *Prenatal and Perinatal Psychology and Medicine–A Comprehensive Survey of Research and Practice,* edited by Peter Feydor-Freyburgh and M. Vogel. New York: Parthenon Publications, 1988.

Van de Carr, R., and M. Lehrer. *The Prenatal Classroom–a Parents' Guide to Teaching Your Baby in the Womb.* Atlanta: Humanics Learning, 1992.

Individualized premature baby care programs

Als, H. A synactive model of neonatal behaviour organisation: a framework for the assessment of neurobehavioral development in the premature infant. *Physical and Occupational Therapy in Paediatrics* 6:3–53, 1986.

——— and F.H.Duffy et al. Earliest Intervention for Preterm Infants in the Newborn Intensive Care Unit. In *The Effectiveness of Early Intervention,* edited by M. J. Guralnick. Baltimore: Baltimore Books, 1997.

Collins, S. K., and K. Kuck. Music therapy in the neonatal intensive care unit. *Neonatal Network* 9(6):23–26, 1991.

Dossey, Barbara, and Lynn Keegan, Cathie E. Guzzetta, and Leslie Kolkmeier. *Holistic Nursing: A Handbook for Practice.* New York:

Aspen Publishers, 1995.

Gerber, Richard. *Vibrational Medicine.* Santa Fe: Bean & Co., 1988.

Als, H., et al. Individualised behavioural and environmental care for the vlbw preterm infant at high risk for BPD: NICU and developmental outcome. *Paediatrics* 78(6):1123–1132, 1986.

———.Individualized behavioral and environmental care for the vlbw preterm infant at high risk of BDP and IVH, study II: NICU Outcome. Abstract, New England Perinatal Association, Woodstock, Vermont:1988.

Als, H., G. Lawhon and F.H. Duffy et al. Individualized behavioral and environmental care of the VLBW infant at high risk for bronchopulmonary dysplasia and intraventricular hemorrhage. *Journal of the American Medical Association*, 272(11), 1994.

Kleberg, A., and B. Westrup et al. Evaluation of the newborn individualised developmental care and assessment program (NIDCAP) in a Swedish setting. *Pediatrics 2000*, 105: 66-72, 1997.

Petryshen, P., et al. Comparing nursing costs for preterm infants receiving conventional vs. developmental care. *Nursing Economics* 15(3), 1997.

Whitley, S., and M. Cowan. Developmental intervention in newborn and intensive care unit. *Clinical Issues in Perinatal and Women's Health Nursing* 2(11):84–110, 1991.

Feeding

Wilson, A. F. Human milk and the pre-term baby. *British Medical Journal*, 306:1628–1629, 1993.

Meier, P. P., and H. H. Mangurten. Breastfeeding the preterm infant. In *Breastfeeding and Human Lactation.* Boston: Jones and Bartlett, 253–278.

Gross, S. J., et al. Nutritional composition of milk produced by mothers delivering preterm. *Journal of Pediatrics* 96: 641–644, 1980.

Mathur, N. B., et al. Anti-infective factors in preterm human colostrum. *Acta Paediatrica Scandinavica* 79:1039–44.

McCain, G. C. Promotion of preterm infant nipple feeding with non-nutrative sucking. *Journal of Pediatric Nursing* 10(1): 3–8, 1995.

Lang, Sandra. *Breastfeeding Special Care Babies.* London: Bailliere Tindall, 1997.

Shaker, C. S. Nipple Feeding

Premature Infants: A Different Perspective. *Neonatal Network* 8 (5): 9–17, 1990.

Steer, P. A., A. Lucas and J. C. Sinclair. Feeding the low birthweight infant. In J. C. Sinclair and M. Bracken (eds.), *Effective Care of the Newborn Infant.* Oxford: Oxford University Press, 1992.

Whitelaw, A., G. Heisterkamp and K. Sleath. Skin to skin contact for very low birthweight infants and their mothers; a randomized trial of kangaroo care. *Archives of Diseases in Childhood* 63: 1377–1381, 1988.

Cues

Blackburn, S. T., and K. A. Vandenburg. Assessment and management of neonatal neurobehavioral development. In C. Kenner, J. W. Lott, A. A. Flandermeyer (eds.), *Comprehensive Neonatal Nursing: A Physiological Perspective.* Philadelphia: W. B. Saunders, 1993.

Carter, Bernadette. Pantomimes of pain, distress, repose and liability: the world of the pre-term baby. *Journal of Child Health Care,* I, Spring l997.

Semmler, Carly J., and Sharon Dowling Butcher. *Handle with Care: Articles about the At-Risk Neonate.* Tucson: Therapy Skill Builders, 1990.

Vandenberg, Kathleen A., and Linda S. Franck. Behavioural issues for infants with BPD. *Neonatal Network* 22, 1990.

COMMON PROBLEMS FOR PREMATURE BABIES

Zaichkin, Jeannette, ed. *Newborn Intensive Care* Petaluma, Ca.:NICU–LINK Publishers, 1997.

SIDS/Apnea connection

American Academy of Pediatrics and American College of Obstetricians and Gynecologists. Postpartum and follow-up care. In *Guidelines for Perinatal Care,* 3rd ed., R.K. Freeman and R.L. Poland (eds.). Elk Grove Village, Illinois: American Academy of Pediatrics, 1996.

Time spent not breathing: how common it is

Glotzbach, S. F., and R. B. Baldwin et al. Periodic breathing in preterm infants: incidence and characteristic. *Pediatrics* 84: 785–792, 1989.

Apnea/bradycardia spells regularly missed in NICUs

Graff, C., and J. Soriano et al. Undetected apnea and bradycardia in infants in special care units (both term and prem). *Pediatric Pulmonology* II:195–7, 1991.

Bradycardia
Hodgman, A., et al. Episodes of bradycardia during early infancy in the term born and pre term infant. *Journal of Diseases of Childhood* 147: 960–964, 1993.

Baby monitors
Levine, J., et al. Report on baby monitors in *Which?* magazine, volume 4 (Feb. 1996) *Science*, Jan. 1999.
Levine, J. et al. Report by Foundation for the Study of Infant Deaths. Nov. 1999.
The National Advisory Board. Third Annual Confidential Enquiry into Stillbirths and Deaths in Infancy. 1996.

Humidity for premature babies with dry, fragile skin
Marshall, Ann. Humidifying the environment for the premature neonate. *Journal of Neonatal Nursing*, Jan. 1977.

Jaundice
Edward, S. Phototherapy and the neonate: Providing safe and effective care for jaundiced infants. *Journal of Neonatal Nursing* 1(5): 9–12, Oct. 1995.

Protecting skull of very low birth-weight baby from pressure induced IVF
Dietch, J. Periventricular–intraventricular haemorrhage in the VLBW infant. *Neonatal Network* 12(1): 7–14, 1993.
Dubowitz, L. and V. *The Neurological Assessment of the Preterm and Full-Term Newborn Infant.* London: Mackeith Press, distributed by Cambridge University Press, first edition 1981, second edition 1999.

MORE SERIOUS PROBLEMS
Fraser Askin, Debbie. Major medical problems. In *Newborn Intensive Care–What Every Parent Needs to Know*, edited by Jeanette Zaichkin. Petaluma, Ca:NICU-LINK Publishers, 1997.
Halliday, Henry. Surfactant therapy: questions and answers. *Journal of Neonatal Nursing* 3 (3): 28–33, May 1997.
Rowe, M. Asphyxiated infants. *Neonatal Network* 9(4) 7–10.
Roberton, N. R. C., editor. *Textbook of Neonatology* New York: Churchill Livingstone, 1986, 1992, 1999.

Intraventricular haemorrhage (IVH)
Periventricular–intraventricular haemorrhage in the very low birth-weight infant. **Neonatal Network** 12(11):7–16.
Kaiser, Anthony. *IVH parents' information leaflet St. Thomas' Hospital,* London, England, n.d.

Eyesight
Gracey, K. M., and K. L. McLaughlin Caring for the infant with retinopathy of prematurity undergoing cryotherapy. *Neonatal Network* 9(7):7–12, 1991.

Lighting
Oehler, J. M. Developmental care of low birth weight infants. *Nursing Clinics of North America* 28(2):289–301, 1993.
Shogan, M. Gordon, and L. L. Schumann. The effect of environmental lighting on the oxygen saturation of preterm infants in the NICU. *Neonatal Network* 12(5):7–13, 1993.

Broncho-pulmonary dysplasia (BDP)
Loftus, John. Medical matters: mechanical ventilation of babies. *Newborn News*, Autumn 1992.

Sedatives making some babies more sensitive to pain
Roberts, R. J. *Drug Therapy in Infants: Pharmacologic Principles and Clinical Experience.* Philadelphia: W. B. Saunders, 1984.
Vandenberg, Katherine A., and Linda S. Frank. Behavioural issues for infants with BPD. *Neonatal Network*, 1990.

MOTHERS
Padden, Tilly, and Sheila Glenn. Maternal experiences of preterm birth and neonatal intensive care. *Journal of Reproductive and Infant Psychology* 15: 121–139, 1997.
Information and Statistics Division. Common Services Agency for the National Health Service, Scotland. Caesarean statistics: 1998 provisional figures.

THE PREMATURE BABY AT HOME
Premature babies' behavior after they leave NICU
Berger, Susan, et al. Caring for the graduate from the neonatal intensive care unit: at home, in the office, and in the community. *Pediatric Clinics of North America* 45(3): 701–12, June 1998.
Fostering family development after preterm hospitalization. In *Pediatric Care of the NICU Graduate*, edited by

R.A. Ballard. Philadelphia: W. B. Saunders, 1988.

How preterm babies' brains and nervous systems develop differently/at different pace than term babies'
Structural and neurobehavioral delay in postnatal brain development of preterm infants. *Pediatric Resources* 39: 895–901, 1996.

Weaning
King, Caroline. Weaning preterm infants onto solids: when, why and how. *The Journal of Neonatal Nursing* 4(6), 1998.

Possible problem areas and their solutions
Blackburn, Susan. Problems of preterm infants after discharge. **Journal of Obstetric, Gynecologic, and Neonatal Nursing** 24: 43–49, Jan. 1995.
Termini, L., et al. Reasons for acute care visits and re-hospitalization in VLBW infants. *Neonatal Network* 8:23–26, 1990.

PREMATURE BABIES: OUTCOMES AND DEVELOPMENT IN THE FIRST FEW YEARS
General
Blackburn, Susan. Problems of preterm infants after discharge. *Journal of Obstetric, Gynecologic, and Neonatal Nursing*, Jan. 1995.
Hack, M., et al. Long term developmental outcomes of low birthweight infants. In Berhman (ed.) *The Future of Children: low birthweight*. Los Altos, California 5(1): Center for the Future of Children, The David and Lucile Packard Foundation, 1995.

Supporting parents of very preterm children
Marlow, Neil, et al. Randomised trial of parental support for families of very preterm children. *Archives of Diseases of Childhood Fetal Neonatal Education* 79:4–11, 1998.

Bright lighting possibly affecting vision
Young, Janine. *Developmental Care of the Premature Baby*. London: Balliere Tindall, 1996.

Noise in NICUs possibly affecting hearing
Letko, M. D. Detecting and preventing infant hearing loss. *Neonatal Network* 1992
Jorgensen, K. M. *Developmental Care of the Premature Infant: A Precise Overview*. Norwell, Massachusetts: Children's Medical Ventures, 1993.

Growth

Manser, J. L. Growth in the high risk neonate. *Clinics in Perinatology* 11:19–40, 1984.

IQ levels

Escobar, G., and B. Littenberg et al. Outcome among surviving very low birthweight infants: a meta analysis. *Archives of Diseases in Childhood* 66: 201–211, 1991.

Hearing

Hack, M., et al. Long term developmental outcomes of low birthweight infants. In Berhman (ed.) *The Future of Children: low birthweight*. Los Altos, California 5(1): Center for the Future of Children, The David and Lucile Packard Foundation, 1995.

Sight

Teplin, S. W., et al. Neurodevelopment health and growth status at age 6 years of children with birth weight of less than 1001g. *Journal of Pediatrics* 118: 768–777, 1991.

Learning problems at school

Bernbaum, S. T., and M. Hoffman-Williamson. *Primary Care of the Preterm Infant*. St. Louis:Mosby Year Book, 1991.

Ornstein, M., and A. Ohlsson et al. Neonatal follow-up of low birthweight/extremely low birthweight infants to school age: a critical overview. *Acta Paediatrica Scandinavica* 80: 741–748 1991.

Saigal, S., et al. Intellectual and functional status at school entry of children who weighed 1000g or less at birth: a regional perspective of birth in the 1980s. *Journal of Pediatrics* 116: 409–416, 1990.

PREMATURITY: CAUSES AND FUTURE PREVENTION

Morrison, J. Clinical, scientific and ethical aspects of fetal and neonatal care at extremely preterm periods of gestation. *British Journal of Obstetrics and Gynaecology* 104, Dec. 1997.

Cervical stitches

Aarts, J. M., et al. Emergency cervical cerclage. *Obstetrics and Gynaecology*, 1995.

MacDougall, J., et al. Emergency cervical cerclage. *British Journal of Obstetrics & Gynaecology* 98, 1991.

Antibiotics

Hauth, J. C., et al. Reduced incidence of preterm delivery with metronidazole and erythromycin in women with bacterial vaginosis. *New England Journal of Medicine* 333: 1732–36, 1995.

Ritrodine

Montquin, J. M., et al, Canadian Preterm Labor Investigators Group. Treatment of preterm labour with the beta-adrenergic agonist ritrodine. *New England Journal of Medicine* 327: 308–12, 1992.

Corticosteroids

Crowley, P. Corticosteroids prior to preterm delivery. In J. P. Neilson et. al (eds.), *Pregnancy & Childbirth Module of The Cochrane Database of Systematic Reviews*. Available in The Cochrane Library, issue 2. Oxford: The Cochrane Collaboration, 1997. www.cochrane.org

Effects of mother's stress levels on baby

Ellis, L., and W. Peckham. Prenatal stress and left-handedness among offspring. *International Journal of Pre and Perinatal Psychology and Medicine* 6 (2): 135–43, Winter 1991.

Glover, V., et al. Association between maternal anxiety during pregnancy and increased uterine artery resistance index: cohort based study. *British Medical Journal* 318 (7177, Jan. 6, l999): 153–7.

Lou, Hans. How Prenatal Stressors for the Mother Affect Foetal Brain Development. Proceedings of the bi-annual meeting of the Marce Society. London, 1996.

Van den Bergh, B. R. H. The influence of maternal emotions during pregnancy on fetal–and neonatal–behaviour. *The International Journal of Pre and Perinatal Psychology and Medicine*, Winter 1990.

War, A. J. Stress and childhood psychopathology. *Child Psychiatry and Human Development* 22:97–110, 1991.

Bradford, Nikki. *The Miraculous World of Your Unborn Baby*. London: Salamander, 2000.

Placental clock/CRH contractions

Smith, R. Alterations in the hypothalamic pituitary adrenal axis during pregnancy and the placental clock that determines the length of parturition. *Journal of Reproductive Immunology* 39(1–2): 215–220, Aug. 1998.

GETTING INFORMATION ON THE INTERNET

There is a wealth of information about prematurity on the Net: possible causes and treatments, the difficulties babies may experience as they grow up, and what can be done to help. There are also details of everything from car seats, clothes and breast pumps, to a vast array of support groups for the parents. Read NET TIPS (below) before proceeding.

MEDLINEplus http://medlineplus.nlm.nih.gov/ From the US National Library of Medicine, the world's biggest database of medical papers, with a variety of useful resources. Pre-prepared searches mean you don't have to worry about the site's complexities and quirks (which are many). Latest medical news and medical dictionaries.

Health on the Net Foundation http://www.hon.ch/ A panel of experts evaluates sites and lists them as either "recommended" or "non-checked" and provides descriptions. Asthma, for example, produces 1,600 unchecked and 64 recommended.

Medical World Search http://www.mwsearch.com/ A bit confusing at first (it has several different settings), but the search engine yields many properly published research papers from high quality medical journals. Worth getting used to if hard, published, clinical info is what you are after.

Medscape http://www.medscape.com/ A site aimed at health professionals with detailed, heavyweight, published clinical papers and research. Very useful if you don't mind the medical terminology.

Healthfinder http://www.healthfinder.org/ Developed by the US Department of Health & Human Services, it helps you find databases, websites, online publications and support groups.

Health Canada http://www.hc-sc.gc.ca/ This bilingual government site yields a wealth of up-to-date, detailed information.

Canadian Health Portal http://www.chp-pcs.gc.ca/ links you to dozens of health sites.

Canadian Health Network http://www.canadian-health-network.ca/ is a collaboration among Health Canada and health organizations and links you to 12,000+ web-based resources. Highly accessible. Bilingual.

Prematurity.org http://www.prematurity.org/ hosts a listserv and a forum for online discussion with neonatologists, health professionals and parents. Research, advocacy and publications.

National Health Information Center http://www.health.gov/ Referral service links consumers to organizations best able to help.

Bright Futures http://www.brightfutures.org/ provides parents and caregivers with up-to-date information on infants, children and adolescents.

Maternal and Child Health Bureau http://www.mchb.hrsa.gov/ has links to government and independent organizations and websites.

NET TIPS

If you are not online at home or work, there are pay-as-you-go cafés and internet centers (with helpful staff to get you started on your Net searches) and many computers linked to the Net in virtually all libraries (where the service is usually free, but often with a wait for a terminal).

Anyone can publish anything on the Net, and they frequently do. So it is worth keeping the following in mind before accepting as a fact any info that you find:

• Who is funding the site? Owner's name(s) should be given along with any sponsorship/advertising deals.

• Is the information up to date? A reliable Web page will state when a piece of info was written and when it was last updated. Be wary of health pages that don't.

• Interesting article—but does it have a named author? If it is written by someone who says they are an expert in this particular subject, run a search on MEDLINE (see above) to see if they have recently had anything on the subject published in a professional peer journal (i.e. where a relevant panel of experts assesses each article or piece of research before they will use it). If they haven't, or if there doesn't seem to be any author that you can see, be wary.

• Ignore anything offering "miracle/wonder cures."

• Or anything that is only backed up by "delighted customer" testimonials rather than published clinical research carried out by someone *other than* the company selling the product.

CARING FOR YOUR CHILD

Neonatalogist

Pediatrician

Nurse practitioner

Pediatric surgeon

Pharmacist

Respiratory therapist

Staff nurses

YOU AND YOUR PREMATURE BABY

Chaplain

Nutritionist

Social worker

Occupational therapist

Physiotherapist

Lactation consultant

Clinical psychologist

Audiologist

Pediatric radiologist

IMPORTANT SPECIALIST SUPPORTING PLAYERS

Pediatric neurologist

Pediatric ophthalmologist

Pediatric cardiologist

Community nurse

Hospital pediatrician

Nurse practitioner

Occupational therapist

Developmental practitioner

YOU AND YOUR GROWING CHILD

Genetics department

Pediatric neurologist

Physiotherapist

Speech therapist

Health visitor nurse

Pediatric ophthalmologist

General practitioner

Pediatric audiologist

Neonatalogist

HELPLINES AND SUPPORT GROUPS

PREMATURITY: WHY DOES IT HAPPEN AND WHAT CAN BE DONE?

Preeclampsia Foundation,
P.O. Box 52993, Bellevue, WA 98015-2993. Helpline 1-800-665-9341
Web www.preeclampsia.org

Best Start Resource Centre 1900-180
Dundas St W, Toronto ON M5G 1Z8
Helpline 1-800-397-9567
Web www.beststart.org
Promotes maternal and newborn health.

Motherisk
The Hospital for Sick Children 555
University Ave, Toronto ON M5G 1X8
Helpline (416) 813-6780.
Web www.motherisk.org.
Info on safety or risk of drugs, chemicals, disease, infection, and radiation exposure during pregnancy and lactation.

March of Dimes
Box 1657, Wilkes-Barres, PA 18703
Helpline 1-888-663-4637
Web www. modimes.com
Helpline staffed by specialists.

Canadian Cancer Society
Suite 200, 10 Alcorn Ave
Toronto ON M4V 3B1
Helpline 1-888-939-3333
Web www.cancer.ca
Free "One Step at a Time" booklet offers support and tips to quit smoking.

American Cancer Society
P.O. Box 102454
Atlanta, GA 20268-2454
Helpline 1-800-ACS-2345
Web www.cancer.org

American Diabetes Association
1701 N. Beauregard St
Alexandria VA 22311
Helpline 1-800-806-7801
Web www.diabetes.org

Canadian Diabetes Association
15 Toronto St., Suite 800
Toronto ON M5C 2E3
Helpline 1-800-banting
Web www.diabetes.ca

The Center for Study of Multiple Birth
Suite 464, 333 E Superior St
Chicago IL 60611
Helpline (312) 908-7532
Web www.multiplebirth.com
Helps parents with problems encountered in multiple births.

Multiple Births Canada
P.O. Box 234, Gormley, ON L0H 1G0
Helpline (905) 888-0725
Web www.multiplebirthscanada.org
Support for multiple birth families and individuals.

National Domestic Violence Hotline (U.S.)
1-800-799-SAFE (7233) 24 Hours
TTY 1-800-787-3224
Web www.ndvh.org
Trained counselors provide crisis assistance and information about shelters, legal advocacy and health care.

National Domestic Violence Hotline (Canada)
Helpline 1-800-363-9010
Bilingual, 24-hour assistance.

Health Canada, Office of
Nutrition Policy and Promotion, Main StatsCanada Building, Room 2701, Tunney's Pasture, AL 0302D
Ottawa, ON K1A 0K9
Helpline (613) 957-8329
Web www.hc-sc.gc.ca/hppb/nutrition
Nutrition for a healthy pregnancy.

Division of Nutrition and Physical Activity, Centers for Disease Control and Prevention
4770 Buford Hwy NE, MS/K-24
Atlanta GA 30341-3717
Fax 1-888-232-4674
Tel (770) 488-5820
Web www.cdc.gov/nccdphp/dnpa
Nutrition tips for pregnancy.

Canadian Health Network
Helpline 1-877- 327-4636
Web www.canadian-health-network.ca
Extensive information and resources on substance abuse in pregnancy.

WHAT CAN WE DO?

Kangaroo Care
The book *Kangaroo Care: The Best You Can Do to Help Your Preterm Infant* by Susan Luddington-Hoe et al is a useful guide.

Homeopathy
To find a homeopath, contact the **North American Society of Homeopaths**, 1122 East Pike Street, Seattle, WA 98122
Helpline (206) 720-7000
Fax (208) 248-1942
Web www.homeopathy.org

Feeding
La Leche League International
P.O. Box 4079
Schaumburg IL 60168-4079
Helpline (847) 519-7730
Fax (847) 519-0035
Web www.lalecheleague.org
Supportive information, products and advocacy. Contact to find a local branch. Some services available in Spanish.

American Cleft Palate-Craniofacial Association/Cleft Palate Foundation
104 South Estes Dr, Suite 204
Chapel Hill, NC 27514
Helpline (919) 933-9044
Web www.cleftline.org

YOU AND YOUR FAMILY
According to the Association for Post-Natal Illness, mothers who have their babies prematurely run a far higher risk of developing some degree of postpartum depression than mothers who have their babies at term. For information, including an online Postpartum Self-Assessment Test and referrals to local support groups and treatment, contact:

Postpartum Support, International
927 North Kellogg Ave
Santa Barbara, CA 93111
Helpline (805) 967-7636
Web www.chss.iup.edu/postpartum
International non-profit organization sponsored by Indiana University of Pennsylvania. Website has worldwide listings of support groups.

La Leche League International (see *Feeding* above)

International Cesarean Awareness Network
1304 Kingsdale Av
Redondo Beach, CA 90278
Helpline (310) 542-6400
Fax (310) 542-5368
Web www.ican-online.org
40 chapters in U.S. and Canada offer education, support and advocacy of a positive recovery from Cesarean birth and option of a vaginal birth after Cesarean (VBAC).

TIME TO GO HOME

Association des parents d'enfants prématuré du Québec
4837, rue Boyer, suite 238
Montréal, QC H2J 3E6
Helpline (514) 523-3974
Fax (514) 523-4167
Web www.colba.net/~apep
English and French-language support group.

Older brothers and sisters
Umass Memorial Medical Center NICU recommends a number of books for siblings, including *I Know I Made It Happen: Children and Guilt* by Lynn Blackburn, *Katie's Premature Brother* by Elizabeth Hawkins-Walsh and *Where's Jess* by Joy Johnson et al, all of which are available at your local library or through Centering Corporation, 1531 Saddle Creek Road, Omaha, NE 68104,
Tel (402) 553-1200,
Fax 402-553-0507
Web www.centering.org

Clothing and home equipment for premature babies
Ask NICU staff and organizations such as La Leche League for recommendations about the necessities and useful items. If you can't find an item locally but do find it online, remember the rules of shopping on the Web: know the company you're dealing with; use secure sites only; *never* send credit details by Email; read the fine print for shipping costs, return policies, and guarantees; and, as always, buyer beware.

La Leche League International (see *Feeding* above)

Baby slings offer convenience and the continual body contact that is important for all babies and particularly premature babies. There are a wide variety of slings and tubes available, most being modern interpretations of the fabric wraps used by traditional cultures worldwide. They allow parents to carry a baby close to the body for long periods of time and can make it easy to nurse discretely. Some are more suitable than others for a smaller baby. To choose what's right for you, seek out consumer reviews in parenting magazines and Websites and talk to other parents for recommendations.
Diapers are widely available in smaller

sizes both in cloth and disposable and recyclable formats, and any reputable diaper service should offer the option of smaller diapers.

SIDS (Crib death)
The Canadian Foundation for the Study of Infant Deaths
Suite 308, 586 Eglinton Ave E
Toronto, ON, M4P 1P2
Helpline 1-800-END-SIDS
Fax (416) 488-3864
Web www.sidscanada.org
National Institute of Child Health and Human Development, Bldg 31, Room 2A32, MSC 2425, 31 Center Drive, Bethesda, MD 20892-2425
Helpline 1-800-505-CRIB (2742)
Web www.nichd.nih.gov/sids/
Information about the "Back to Health" campaign (see page 172).
National Sudden Infant Death Syndrome Resource Center
2070 Chain Bridge Rd, Suite 450, Vienna, VA 22182
Helpline (703) 821-8955
Fax (703) 821-2098
Web www.sidscenter.org
Information and support for parents regarding SIDS, apnea, bereavement and more. Publishes *The Death of a Child— The Grief of the Parents: A Lifetime Journey* available online or by mail.

General Child Care
Healthfinder
P.O. Box 1133
Washington, DC 20013-1133
Web www.healthfinder.gov
Operating since 1997 as a key resource for finding government and nonprofit health information. Links to information and Web sites from over 1800 health-related organizations. Also in Spanish.
National Child Care Information Center
243 Church St NW 2nd Floor
Vienna, VA 22180
Helpline 1-800-616-2242
TTY 1-800-516-2242
Fax 1-800-716-2242
Web www.nccic.org
Created in partnership with Child Care Bureau, Administration for Children and Families, US Department of Health and Human Services, and the University of Illinois at Urbana-Champaign. Information on childcare resources in your state as well as links to various other childcare-related organizations. Also in Spanish.

SPECIAL BABIES, SPECIAL CHILDREN
National Information Center for Children and Youth with Disabilities
P.O. Box 1492
Washington, DC 20013
Helpline 1-800-695-0285
TTY 1-800-695-0285
Fax (202) 884-8441
Web www.nichcy.org
A good place to start to find information and assistance about disabilities. Free

online and printed publications, assistance connecting with local resources and a toll-free helpline. Also in Spanish.
Cerebral Palsy
The National Institute of Neurological Disorders and Stroke
National Institutes of Health
Bethesda, MD 20892
Helpline 1-800-352-9424
TTY (301) 468-5981
Web www.ninds.nih.gov
Information and links to other support groups.
United Cerebral Palsy National
1660 L Street NW, Suite 700
Washington, DC 20036
Helpline 1-800-872-5827
TTY (202) 973-7197
Fax 202-776-0414
Web www.ucpa.org
Principal non-government agency sponsoring research to prevent cerebral palsy and improve the quality of life.
Ontario Federation for Cerebral Palsy
104-1630 Lawrence Ave W
Toronto ON M6L 1C5
Helpline 1-877-244-9686
Fax (416) 244-6543
Better resources than the national site, and with links to provincial bodies. *A Guide to Cerebral Palsy* publication is a good place to start. It has recommended reading and where to find more information.
American Society for Deaf Children,
P.O. Box 3355, Gettysburg, PA 17325
Helpline/TTY (717) 334-7922
Fax (717) 334-8808
Web www.deafchildren.org
The Canadian Hearing Society
271 Spadina Road
Toronto, ON M5R 2V3
Helpline (416) 964-9595
TTY (416) 964-0023
Fax (416) 928-2525
Web www.chs.ca
National organization offers American Sign Language classes, audiology services and speech therapy, hearing aid sales, interpretation, counseling, advocacy and public education.
American Lung Association
61 Broadway, 6th Floor
New York, NY 10006
Helpline (212) 315-8700
Web www.lungusa.org
Available in Spanish.
Canadian Lung Association
Helpline 1-888-566-LUNG (5864)
Web www.lung.ca
Asthma Resource Center provides extensive information. Bilingual. Website has list of provincial groups.
Epilepsy Canada
1470 Peel Street, Suite 745
Montreal, PQ H3A 1T1
Helpline 1-877-734-0873
Fax (514) 845-7866
Web www.epilepsy.ca
Epilepsy Foundation
4351 Garden City Drive
Landover, MD 20785-7223

Helpline 1-800-332-1000
Web www.efa.org
Online zip-code locator helps you find local services.
ADHD/LD
National Institute of Mental Health,
NIMH Public Inquiries
6001 Executive Blvd
Rm 8184, MSC 9663,
Bethesda, MD 20892-9663
Helpline (301) 443-4513
Fax (301) 443-4279
Web www.nimh.nih.gov
Various publications on Attention Deficit Hyperactivity Disorder and Learning Disorders available online or for a nominal fee.
Spina Bifida Association of America
Information & Referral Dept.
4590 MacArthur Blvd NW
Suite 250, Washington, DC 20017-4226
Helpline (202) 944-3285.
www.sbaa.org
Online directories list local chapters and clinics across USA. Many documents available online.
Spina Bifida and Hydrocephalus Association of Canada
977–167 Lombard Ave
Winnipeg MB R3B 0V3
Helpline 1-800-565-9488
Fax (204) 925-3654
Web www.sbhac.ca

GRIEVING AND LOSS
SHARE
St. Joseph Health Center
300 First Capitol Dr
St. Charles, MO 63301-2893
Helpline 1-800-821-6819
Fax (636) 947-7486
Web nationalshareoffice.com
Non-denominational organization offers support to those who have suffered the loss of a baby. All services and publications are free.
Bereaved Families of Ontario
36 Eglinton Ave W, Suite 602
Toronto, ON M4R 1A1
Helpline (416) 440-0290
Fax (416) 440-0304
Web www.bereavedfamilies.net
Support tailored to individual needs with special groups for parents of infants, plus for toddlers, children, adolescents, young adults and grandparents.
Bereaved Parents of the USA
PO Box 95
Park Forest, IL 60466
Fax (708) 748-9184
Web www.bereavedparentsusa.org
Non-profit, voluntary organization aims to educate families about the grief process and to provide emotional support. Branches have libraries of reading material, and members offer support to the newly bereaved.

See also, *Getting Information on the Internet* on page 202.

index

Page numbers in *italics* indicate illustrations.

Publishers' acknowledgments

The impulse to produce this book stemmed from the life of a baby who is very special to us: Gianni Litchmore Bonfanti, who was born on 3 July 1997, at 27 weeks, and lived for nine weeks.

Commissioning Editor Jo Christian
Editor Sarah Mitchell
Editorial help Michael Brunström, Judith Warren
Index Tarrant Ranger Indexing

Art Editor Louise Kirby
Designer Becky Clarke
Art Director Caroline Hillier

Production Hazel Kirkman

Photographic acknowledgments

All photographs copyright © Sandra Lousada, except for those otherwise indicated, and the following:
© Sam Richards pages 19, 31, 91
© Martin Sharratt pages 103, 143
© Pauline Sharratt page 63
The photograph on page 67 was taken by a nurse in Kingston Hospital.
Sandra Lousada would like to say that, although she took the great majority of the photographs that appear in this book, the two photographs she considers the best were not taken by her or by any professional photographer, but by parents. Sam Richards took the photograph of Ellen on page 19, and Martin Sharratt took the photograph of Isabel and John on page 103; she hopes this will inspire parents to take and value their own pictures of their children.
We are very grateful to all the parents who allowed us to photograph their babies for this book. Special thanks to the parents of: Simone and Amber Eakins, Joseph Edu, Ella and George Ewart, Gabrielle Fulgoni, Elizabeth Hackney, Emily Grace Hale, Tom, Ben and Megan Hughes-Jones, Aaron Jarvis, Ryan Munday, Baby Namwenda, Archie, Storm and Imogen Parrish, Alec Sargood, George Schiessl, John Sharratt, Nina and Ellen Taurich, and Matthew Withington.
We also wish to thank St Thomas's Hospital, London, Kingston Hospital NHS Trust, Surrey and Santa Monica Hospital UCLA, who gave us permission to take photographs in their Special Care Baby Units, and Nurse Bada and Nurse Beverley who allowed us to photograph them.